KETO AIR FRYER COOKBOOK

Healthy and Easy Delicious Recipes for Smart People

(Easy and Affordable Recipes to Lose Weight Quickly)

Velma Perry

Published by Sharon Lohan

© **Velma Perry**

All Rights Reserved

Keto Air Fryer Cookbook: Healthy and Easy Delicious Recipes for Smart People (Easy and Affordable Recipes to Lose Weight Quickly)

ISBN 978-1-7776245-8-3

All rights reserved. No part of this guide may be reproduced in any form without permission in writing from the publisher except in the case of brief quotations embodied in critical articles or reviews.

Legal & Disclaimer

The information contained in this book is not designed to replace or take the place of any form of medicine or professional medical advice. The information in this book has been provided for educational and entertainment purposes only.

The information contained in this book has been compiled from sources deemed reliable, and it is accurate to the best of the Author's knowledge; however, the Author cannot guarantee its accuracy and validity and cannot be held liable for any errors or omissions. Changes are periodically made to this book. You must consult your doctor or get professional medical advice before using any of the suggested remedies, techniques, or information in this book.

Table of contents

Part 1 1
1. Bacon Avocado Fries 2
2. Cauliflower Tots 4
3. Air Fryer Steak 7
4. Air Fryer Salmon 9
5. Brussels Sprout Chips 10
6. Air Fryer Rotisserie Chicken 13
7. Crispy Air Fryer Bacon 15
8. Apple Chips 16
9. Air Fryer Thanksgiving Turkey 18
10. Air Fryer Spicy Chicken Thighs 20
11. Buffalo Chicken Keto Cauliflower Tots 22
12. KETO AIR FRYER MEATLOAF SLIDERS 24
13. KETOAIR FRYER BAKED CHICKEN NUGGETS 27
14. Fried Cheesecake Bites 30
15. Keto Air Fryer Fish Sticks 32
16. KETO COCONUT SHRIMP 34
17. KETO CREAMED SPINACH 37
18. Keto Jalapeno Poppers 39
19. AIR FRYER ROASTED BRUSSELS SPROUTS 41
20. AIR FRIED CAULIFLOWER RICE 43
21. Keto Air Fryer Chickpeas 45
22. Air Fryer Steak Bites and Mushrooms 47
23. Tomato Basil Scallops 49
25. AIR FRYER ONION RINGS 54

Part 2	57
Introduction	58
Chapter 1	59
Ketogenic Diets And Their Rapid Weight Loss Effects	59
Chapter 2	64
5 Tips For Success on the Ketogenic Diet	64
Chapter 3	69
Category of Foods To Consume on Ketogenic Diet	69
Chapter 4: Delicious Air-Fryer Recipes	73
1. Eggs & Diary	73
Bacon & Egg Bite Cups	73
Avocado With Eggs & Bacon	76
Baked Egg Cups Spinach & Cheese	78
Bacon, Egg and Cheese Roll-Ups	80
Scrambled Eggs	82
Scotch Eggs	84
Baked Potted Egg	86
2. Beef Recipe	88
Meatloaf Sliders	88
3. Sea Foods	90
Coconut Shrimp	90
Fish Sticks	93
Crab Cakes	95
Tomato Mayonnaise Shrimp	97
4. Vegetables	99
Delicious Roasted Veggies	99
Zucchini Pizza Boats	101

Sausage Balls	103
Cauliflower With Buffalo Sauce	105
Spinach & Artichoke Dip	108
Creamed Spinach	110
Breakfast Casserole	111
Stuffed Peppers	114
Breakfast Frittata	115
5. Chicken Recipes	118
Crispy Chicken Wings	118
Tandoori Chicken Recipe	120
Crispy Chicken Nuggets	122
Herb-Marinated Chicken Thighs	124
Popcorn Chicken	126
Greek Chicken Stir-Fry	128
Parmesan Chicken Meatballs	129
6. Pork Recipes	131
Breakfast Sausage	131
Crispy Pork Chops	133
Pork Chops & Broccoli	134
Pork Chops With Brown Butter & Sage	136
Bacon Wrapped Jalapeno Poppers	138
Low Carb Zucchini Fries	140
Fried Cheesecake Bites	142
Avocado Fries	143
Mozzarella Sticks	145
Delicious Rolls	149
Air Fryer Biscuits	151

Air Fry Olive Bread 153
Lunch & Dinner Recipes 155
1. Chicken Recipes 155
Chicken Thighs With Adobo Seasoning 155
Buttermilk Fried Chicken 156
Gochujang Chicken Wings (Korean Recipe) 158
Chicken Wings With Sauce 161
4-Ingredients Keto Wings 164
Chicken Hot Wings With Buffalo Sauce 165
Whole Chicken Recipe 168
Spicy Dry-Rubbed Chicken Wings 170
Cornish Hens Recipe 172
Almond Flour Air Fried Chicken 174
Garlic Parmesan Chicken Wings 176
Lemon-Garlic Chicken Thighs 178
Chicken & Broccoli 180
Southern-Style Chicken Recipe 182
5 – Ingredient Crispy & Cheesy Dinner Chicken 183
Pizza Stuffed Chicken 186

Part 1

1. Bacon Avocado Fries

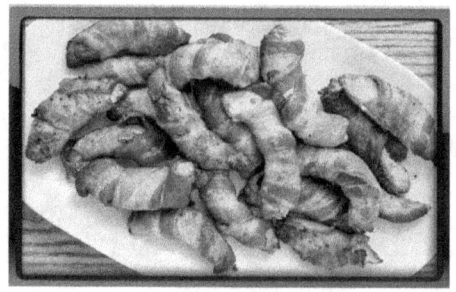

Serving=2

Cooking time =5 minutes

INGREDIENTS

- 3 avocados
- 24 thin strips of bacon
- 1/4 c. ranch dressing, for serving

DIRECTIONS

FOR OVEN

1. Preheat oven to 425º. Slice every avocado into eight equally-sized wedges. Wrap every wedge in bacon, reducing bacon if needed. Place on a baking sheet, seam aspect down.
2. Bake till bacon is cooked thru and crispy, 12 to fifteen minutes.
3. Serve with ranch dressing.

FOR AIR FRYER

1. Slice every avocado into eight equally-sized wedges. Wrap every wedge with a strip of bacon, slicing bacon if needed.
2. Working in batches, set up in air fryer basket in a unmarried layer. Cook at 400° for eight mins till bacon is cooked thru and crispy.
3. SERVE HOT WITH RANCH.

2. Cauliflower Tots

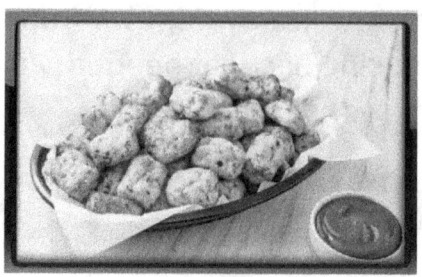

SERVING=6

COOKING TIME = 30 MINUTES

INGREDIENTS

- Cooking spray
- 4 c. cauliflower florets, steamed (about 1/2 large cauliflower)
- 1 large egg, lightly beaten
- 1 c. shredded cheddar
- 1 c. freshly grated Parmesan
- 2/3 c. panko breadcrumbs
- 2 tbsp. freshly chopped chives

- Kosher salt
- Freshly ground black pepper
- 1/2 c. ketchup
- 2 tbsp. Sriracha

DIRECTIONS

FOR OVEN

1. Preheat oven to 375°. Grease a massive baking sheet with cooking spray.

2. In a meals processor, pulse steamed cauliflower till riced. Place riced cauliflower on a smooth kitchen towel and squeeze to empty water.

3. Transfer cauliflower to a massive bowl with egg, cheddar, Parmesan, Panko, and chives and blend till combined. Season with salt and pepper to taste.

4. Spoon approximately 1 tablespoon aggregate and roll it right into a tater-tot form together along with your hands. Place on organized baking sheet and bake for 15 to twenty minutes, till children are golden.

5. Meanwhile, make highly spiced ketchup: Combine ketchup and Sriracha in a small serving bowl and stir to combine.

6. Serve heat cauliflower children with highly spiced ketchup.

FOR AIR FRYER

7. In a meals processor, pulse steamed cauliflower till riced. Place riced cauliflower on a easy kitchen towel and squeeze to empty water.

8. Transfer cauliflower to a big bowl with egg, cheddar, Parmesan, Panko, and chives and blend till combined. Season with salt and pepper to taste.

9. Spoon approximately 1 tablespoon aggregate and roll it right into a tater-tot form together along with your hands. Working in batches, set up in basket of air fryer in a unmarried layer and prepare dinner dinner at 375° for 10, till toddlers are golden.

10. Meanwhile, make highly spiced ketchup: Combine ketchup and Sriracha in a small serving bowl and stir to combine.

11. Serve heat cauliflower toddlers with highly spiced ketchup.

3. Air Fryer Steak

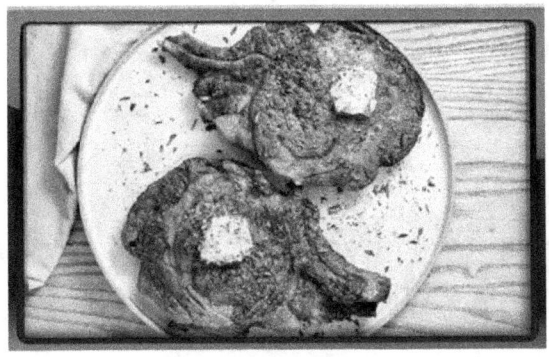

SERVING=2

COOKING TIME = 45 MINUTES

INGREDIENTS

- 4 tbsp. butter, softened
- 2 cloves garlic, minced
- 2 tsp. freshly chopped parsley
- 1 tsp. freshly chopped chives
- 1 tsp. freshly chopped thyme
- 1 tsp. freshly chopped rosemary
- 1 (2 lb.) bone-in ribeye

- Kosher salt

- Freshly ground black pepper

DIRECTIONS

1. In a small bowl, integrate butter and herbs. Place in middle of a chunk of plastic wrap and roll right into a log. Twist ends collectively to hold tight and refrigerate till hardened, 20 minutes.

2. Season steak on each facets with salt and pepper.

3. Place steak in basket of air fryer and prepare dinner dinner at 400° for 12 to fourteen minutes, for medium, relying on thickness of steak, flipping midway through.

4. Top steak with a slice of herb butter to serve.

4. Air Fryer Salmon

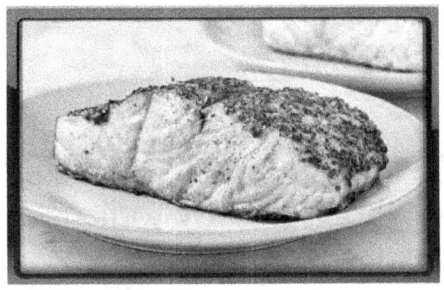

SERVING=2

COOKING TIME = 15 MINUTES

INGREDIENTS

- 2 (6-oz.) salmon fillets
- Kosher salt
- Freshly ground black pepper
- 2 tsp. extra-virgin olive oil
- 2 tbsp. whole grain mustard
- 1 tbsp. packed brown sugar
- 1 clove garlic, minced
- 1/2 tsp. thyme leaves

DIRECTIONS

1. Season salmon throughout with salt and pepper. In a small bowl, whisk collectively oil, mustard, sugar, garlic, and thyme. Spread on pinnacle of salmon.

2. Arrange salmon in air fryer basket. Set air fryer to 400° and prepare dinner dinner for 10 minutes.

5.Brussels Sprout Chips

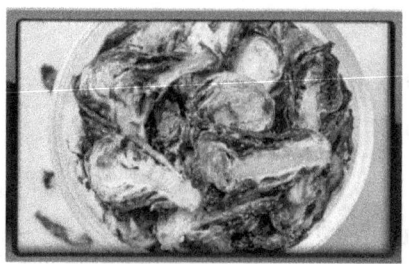

SERVING= 2-3

COOKING TIME = 25 MINUTES

INGREDIENTS

- 1/2 lb. brussels sprouts, thinly sliced
- 1 tbsp. extra-virgin olive oil
- 2 tbsp. freshly grated Parmesan, plus more for garnish
- 1 tsp. garlic powder
- Kosher salt
- Freshly ground black pepper
- Caesar dressing, for dipping

DIRECTIONS

FOR OVEN

1. Preheat oven to 400°. In a huge bowl, toss brussels sprouts with oil, Parmesan, and garlic powder and season with salt and pepper. Spread in a fair layer on a medium baking sheet.
2. Bake 10 mins, toss, and bake eight to ten mins extra, till crisp and golden. Garnish with extra

Parmesan and serve with caesar dressing for dipping.

FOR AIR FRYER

3. In a massive bowl, toss brussels sprouts with oil, Parmesan, and garlic powder and season with salt and pepper. Arrange in a fair layer in air fryer.
4. Bake at 350° for eight mins, toss, and bake eight mins extra, till crisp and golden.
5. Garnish with extra Parmesan and serve with caesar dressing for dipping. And your recipe is ready

6. Air Fryer Rotisserie Chicken

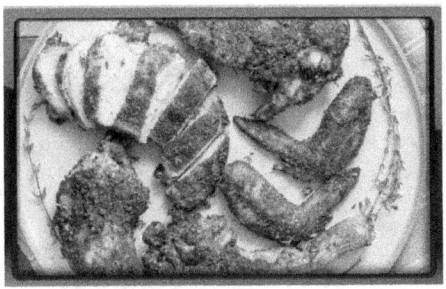

SERVING= 6

COOKING TIME =1 Hour 10 MINUTES

INGREDIENTS

- 1 (3-lb) chicken, cut into 8 pieces
- Kosher salt
- Freshly ground black pepper
- 1 tbsp. dried thyme
- 2 tsp. dried oregano
- 2 tsp. garlic powder
- 2 tsp. onion powder

- 1 tsp. smoked paprika
- 1/4 tsp. Cayenne

DIRECTIONS

1. Season hen portions throughout with salt and pepper. In a medium bowl, whisk to mix herbs and spices, then rub spice blend throughout hen portions.
2. Add darkish meat portions to air fryer basket and prepare dinner dinner at 350° for 10 mins, then turn and prepare dinner dinner 10 mins more.
3. Repeat with chook breasts, however decreasing time to eight mins in step with side. Use a meat thermometer to insure that chook is cooked through, every piece must sign in 165°.

7. Crispy Air Fryer Bacon

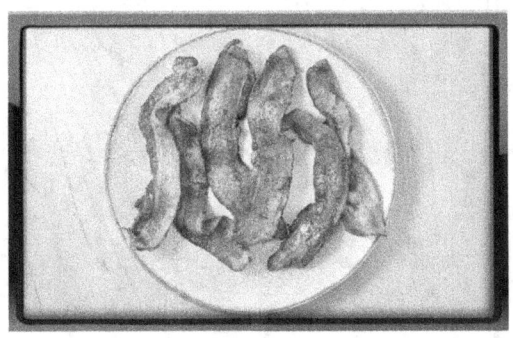

SERVING= 1-2

COOKING TIME = 15 MINUTES

INGREDIENTS

- 3/4 lb. thick-cut bacon

DIRECTIONS

1. Lay bacon interior air fryer basket in a unmarried layer.

2. Set air fryer to 400° and prepare dinner dinner till crispy, approximately 10 minutes. (You can take a look at midway via and rearrange slices with tongs.)

8.Apple Chips

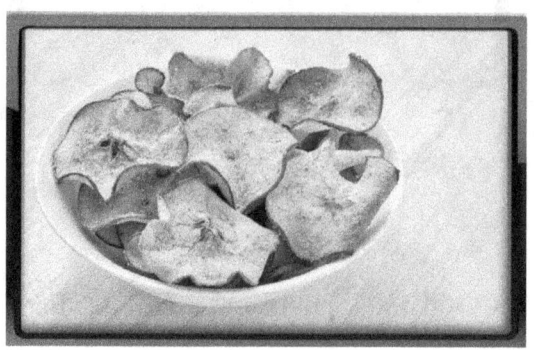

SERVING= 2

COOKING TIME = 3 Hours

INGREDIENTS

- 2 apples, thinly sliced
- 2 tsp. granulated sugar
- 1/2 tsp. Cinnamon

DIRECTIONS

FOR OVEN

1. Preheat oven to 200°. In a massive bowl, toss apples with sugar and cinnamon.
2. Place a metallic rack interior a rimmed baking sheet. Lay apples slices on pinnacle of rack, spacing them in order that no apples overlap.
3. Bake for two to a few hours, flipping apples midway through, till apples dried out however nevertheless pliable. (Apples will preserve to crisp at the same time as cooling.)

FOR AIR FRYER

4. In a big bowl toss apples with cinnamon and sugar. Working in batches, area apples in a unmarried layer in basket of air fryer (a few overlap is okay).
5. Bake at 350° for approximately 12 minutes, flipping each four minutes.

9. Air Fryer Thanksgiving Turkey

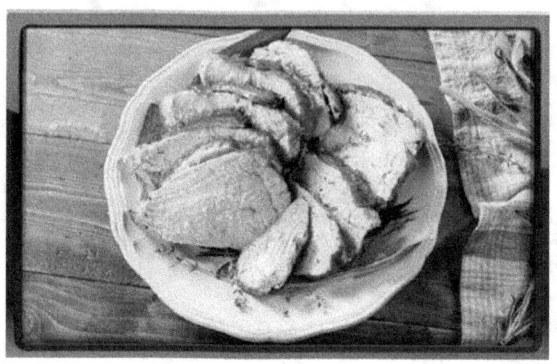

SERVING= 4

COOKING TIME = 1 Hour

INGREDIENTS

- 1 (2-lb.) turkey breast
- Kosher salt
- Freshly ground black pepper
- 1 tsp. freshly chopped thyme
- 1 tsp. freshly chopped rosemary

- 1 tsp. freshly chopped sage
- 1/4 c. maple syrup
- 2 tbsp. dijon mustard
- 1 tbsp. butter, melted

DIRECTIONS

1. Season turkey breast generously with salt and pepper, then rub throughout with clean herbs.
2. Place in air fryer and fry at 390º for 30 to 35 mins or till the inner temperature reaches 160º.
3. In a small bowl, whisk collectively maple syrup, dijon, and melted butter.
4. Remove turkey from air fryer and brush combination throughout. Return to air fryer and fry at 330º till caramelized, 2 mins.
5. Let relaxation 15 mins earlier than slicing.

10. Air Fryer Spicy Chicken Thighs

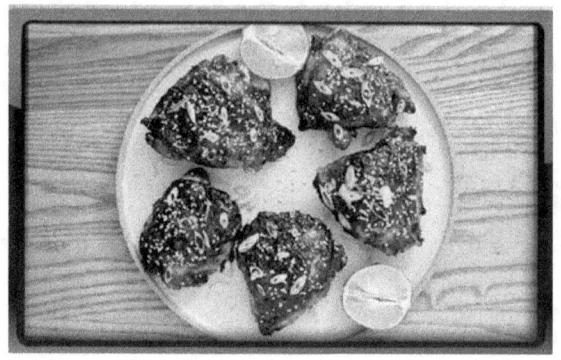

SERVING= 4

COOKING TIME = 1 Hours 20 minutes

INGREDIENTS

- 1/3 c. low-sodium soy sauce
- 1/4 c. extra-virgin olive oil
- 2 tbsp. honey
- 2 tbsp. chili garlic sauce
- Juice of 1 lime

- 2 cloves garlic, minced
- 2 tsp. freshly grated ginger
- 4 bone-in, skin-on chicken thighs (about 2 lb.)
- Thinly sliced green onions, for garnish
- Toasted sesame seeds, for garnish

DIRECTIONS

1. In a big bowl, integrate soy sauce, oil, honey, chili garlic sauce, lime juice, garlic, and ginger. Reserve ½ cup of marinade. Add hen thighs to bowl and toss to coat. Cover and refrigerate for at the least 30 minutes.
2. Remove 2 thighs from marinade and vicinity in basket of air fryer. Cook at 400° till thighs are cooked thru to an inner temperature of 165°, 15 to twenty minutes. Transfer thighs to a plate and tent with foil. Repeat with last thighs.
3. Meanwhile, in a small saucepan over medium warmth, convey reserved marinade to a boil. Reduce warmth and simmer till sauce thickens slightly, four to five minutes.
4. Brush sauce over thighs and garnish with inexperienced onions and sesame seeds earlier than serving.

11. Buffalo Chicken Keto Cauliflower Tots

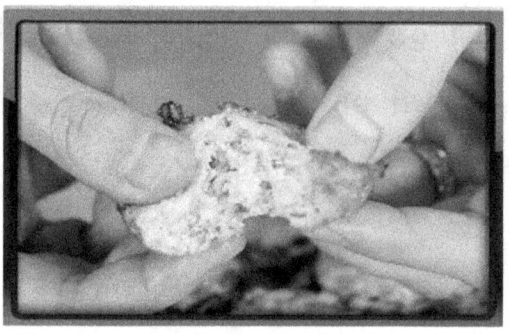

SERVING= 24 tots

COOKING TIME = 15 minutes

Ingredients

- 2 cups Cauliflower
- 1/2 teaspoon Garlic powder
- 8 ounces Rotisserie Seasoned Chicken Breast from Prime Fresh Delicatessen chopped
- 1 egg
- 3/4 cup Parmesan cheese

- 2 Tablespoons Buffalo sauce
- 4 Tablespoons Parmesan cheese
- 6 Tablespoons Almond flour

DIRECTIONS

1. Chop cauliflower into "pearls" the use of a meals processor.
2. Add chopped cauliflower, chopped Prime Fresh Deli Chicken, garlic powder, egg, and 3/four cup Parmesan cheese, and Buffalo sauce to a massive blending bowl.
3. Mix elements collectively till properly combined.
4. Roll aggregate into balls approximately 1 teaspoon in size.
5. In a separate bowl, stir collectively four Tablespoons Parmesan cheese and six Tablespoons almond flour.
6. Gently roll every cauliflower bird ball withinside the coating, then shape into "tater tot" shapes.
7. Add 1/four cup coconut oil to a frying pan or sauté pan. Heat oil over medium heat.

8. Arrange cauliflower little toddlers on their facet in pan, in a single 1/2 of of the pan. (We cooked ours in batches of approximately 6 little toddlers, however this will range primarily based totally on the scale of your pan).

9. Fry cauliflower little toddlers for 2-five minutes, lightly rolling them from one facet of the pan to the other, to make sure that each one facets prepare dinner dinner equally. (This is why we positioned them in simplest 1/2 of of the pan to start).

10. When little toddlers are golden brown, cast off from pan and area on paper towels to cool.

12.KETO AIR FRYER MEATLOAF SLIDERS

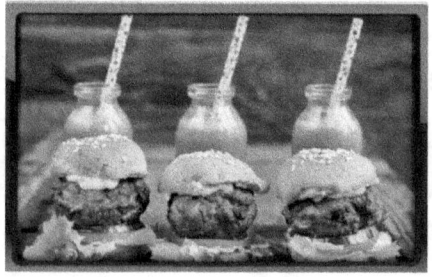

SERVING= 8

COOKING TIME = 20 minutes

Ingredients

- 1 lb ground beef, 80/20 fat
- 2 eggs, beaten
- ¼ C onion, finely chopped
- 1 clove garlic, minced
- ½ C blanched almond flour, extra fine
- ¼ C coconut flour
- ¼ C ketchup
- ½ tsp sea salt
- ½ tsp black pepper
- 1 Tbsp Worcestershire Sauce
- 1 tsp Italian Seasoning, See below
- ½ tsp Tarragon, dried

DIRECTIONS

1. In a big blending bowl, integrate all of the components and blend well. Make patties that are

2. approximately 2" in diameter and approximately 1" thick. If you need to make thicker or thinner patties,

3. ensure they all are comparable in size, in order that they prepare dinner dinner well on the identical time. Place the patties on a platter and refrigerate for 10 mins for the flour to soak up the moist components and the patties to grow to be firm.

4. Preheat the air fryer to 360°F.

5. Place as many patties you could in shape withinside the basket and close. Set the timer for 10 mins.

6. Check the patties 1/2 of way. When the timer is going off, take them out to a serving platter and cowl till all of the patties are cooked.

7. These sliders are ideal in your favourite paleo breads or biscuits (p.164) or on lettuce wraps or with a aspect of spring greens.

13. KETO AIR FRYER BAKED CHICKEN NUGGETS

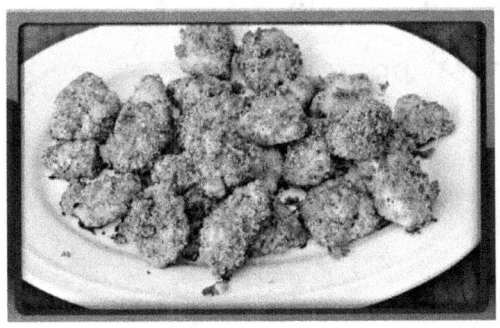

SERVING = 4

COOKING TIME = 25 minutes

Ingredients

- 1 Pound Free-range boneless, skinless chicken breast
- Pinch sea salt
- 1 tsp Sesame oil
- 1/4 Cup Coconut flour
- 1/2 tsp Ground ginger

- 4 Egg whites
- 6 Tbsp Toasted sesame seeds
- Cooking spray of choice

For Dipping

- 2 Tbsp Natural creamy almond butter
- 4 tsp Coconut aminos (or GF soy sauce)
- 1 Tbsp Water
- 2 tsp Rice vinegar
- 1 tsp Sriracha, or to taste
- 1/2 tsp Ground ginger
- 1/2 tsp Monkfruit (omit for whole30)

DIRECTIONS

1. Preheat you air fryer to four hundred levels for 10 mins.

2. While the air fryer heats, reduce the hen into nuggets (approximately 1 inch pieces,) dry them off and location them in a bowl. Toss with salt and sesame oil till lined.

3. Place the coconut flour and floor ginger in a big Ziploc bag and shake to combine. Add the hen and shake till lined.

4. Place the egg whites in a big bowl and upload withinside the hen nuggets, tossing till they may be all properly lined withinside the egg.

5. Place the sesame seeds in a big, Ziploc bag. Shake any extra egg off the hen and upload the nuggets into the bag, shake till properly lined.

6. GENEROUSLY spray the mesh air fryer basket with cooking spray. Place the nuggets into the basket,* ensuring to now no longer crowd them or they won't get crispy. Spray with a hint of cooking spray.

7. Cook for six mins. Flip every nugget and spray for cooking spray. Then, prepare dinner dinner a further 5-6 mins till not red inside, with a crispy outside.

8. While the nuggets prepare dinner dinner, whisk all of the sauce substances collectively in a medium bowl till smooth.

9. Serve the nuggets with the dip and DEVOUR!

14. Fried Cheesecake Bites

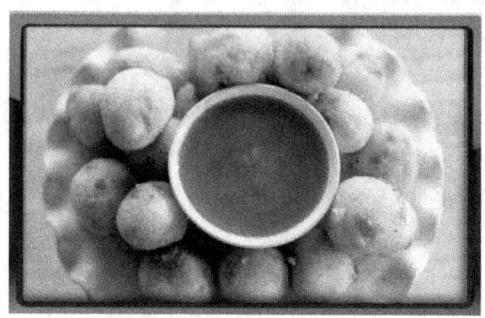

SERVING= 4

COOKING TIME = 25 minutes

Ingredients

- 8 ounces cream cheese
- 1/2 cup erythritol
- 4 Tablespoons heavy cream, divided
- 1/2 teaspoon vanilla extract
- 1/2 cup almond flour
- 2 Tablespoons erythritol

DIRECTIONS

1. Allow the cream cheese to take a seat down at the counter for 20 mins to soften.
2. Fit a stand mixer with paddle attachment.
3. Mix the softened cream cheese, half of cup erithrytol, vanilla and heavy cream till smooth.
4. Scoop onto a parchment paper covered baking sheet.
5. Freeze for approximately 30 mins, till firm.
6. Mix the almond flour with the two Tablespoons erythritol in a small blending bowl.
7. Dip the frozen cheesecake bites into 2 Tablespoons cream, then roll into the almond flour mixture.
8. Place in an air fryer at three hundred levels for two mins.

15. Keto Air Fryer Fish Sticks

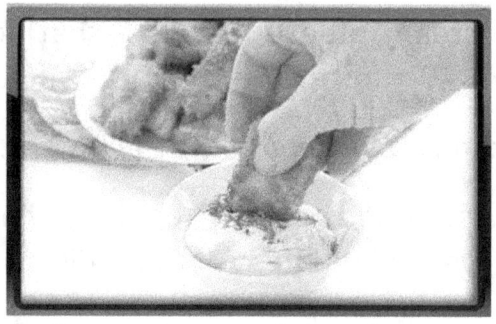

SERVING= 4

COOKING TIME = 20 minutes

Ingredients

- 1 lb white fish such as cod
- 1/4 cup mayonnaise
- 2 tbsp Dijon mustard
- 2 tbsp water
- 1 1/2 cups pork rind panko such as Pork King Good

- 3/4 tsp cajun seasoning
- Salt and pepper to taste

DIRECTIONS

1. Spray the air fryer rack with non-stick cooking spray (I use avocado oil spray).
2. Pat the fish dry and reduce into sticks approximately 1 inch with the aid of using 2 inches huge (how you're capable of reduce it's going to rely a bit on what type of fish you with the aid of using and the way thick and huge it is).
3. In a small shallow bowl, whisk collectively the mayo, mustard, and water. In any other shallow bowl, whisk collectively the red meat rinds and Cajun seasoning. Add salt and pepper to flavor (each the red meat rinds and seasoning ought to have a truthful little bit of salt so dip a finger in to flavor how salty it is).
4. Working with one piece of fish at a time, dip into the mayo aggregate to coat after which faucet off the excess. Dip into the red meat rind aggregate and toss to coat. Place at the air fryer rack.

5. Set to Air Fry at 400F and bake five minutes, the turn the fish sticks with tongs and bake any other five minutes. Serve immediately.

16. KETO COCONUT SHRIMP

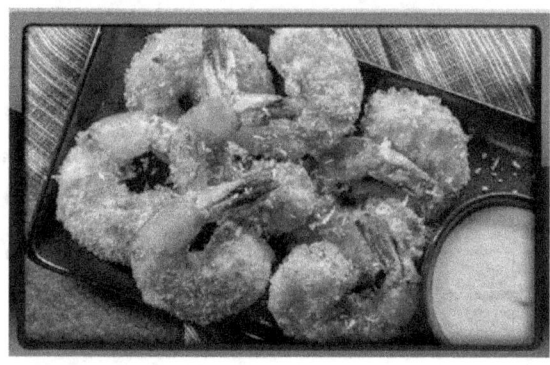

SERVING= 4

COOKING TIME = 20 minutes

Ingredients

- 1/2 lb tail-on large shrimp
- 1 egg, beaten
- 1/2 cup shredded coconut

- 1 tsp garlic powder
- 1/2 tsp paprika
- 1/4 tsp onion powder
- 1/4 tsp salt

DIRECTIONS

1. Place the shredded coconut right into a bowl and blend withinside the garlic powder, paprika, onion powder and salt, after which beat the egg in a one-of-a-kind bowl. Place the bowls subsequent to every other.
2. Use a cooking spray oil to coat the lowest of the air fryer basket.
3. Next, location a shrimp into the bowl with the crushed egg and coat it completely. Transfer it to the bowl with the shredded coconut and coat completely. Immediately location the coconut shrimp into the air fryer basket.
4. Repeat step three till the air fryer basket is complete in a single layer with the shrimp. Shrimp may be barely touching, however don't % them in wonderful tightly. You will want to prepare dinner dinner them in 2 batches.

5. Cook on 350 ranges F. For 10 minutes.

6. While the primary batch cooks, repeat the system with the second one batch, placed location on a plate as soon as every shrimp has been coated.

7. When the air fryer is done, use tongs to cautiously eliminate every shrimp. To without problems eliminate, slip one facet of the tongs below the coconut shrimp first earlier than pulling up and removing.

8. Place on a plate or serving platter, after which upload the second one batch of shrimp and repeat cooking for 10 minutes.

9. Serve with cocktail sauce or Pineapple Thai sauce

17. KETO CREAMED SPINACH

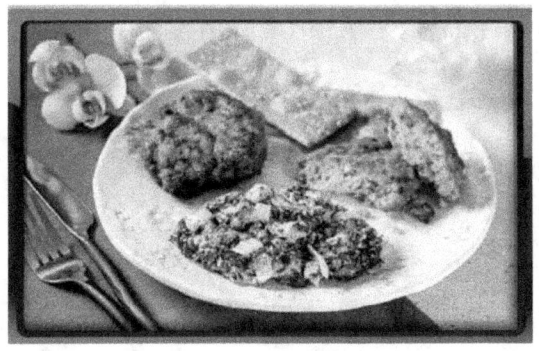

SERVING = 4

COOKING TIME = 20 minutes

Ingredients

- 1 10 ounce package (1 10 ounce package) Frozen Spinach, thawed
- 1/2 cup (80 g) onions, chopped
- 2 teaspoons (2 teaspoons) Minced Garlic
- 4 ounces (113.4 g) Cream Cheese, diced
- 1 teaspoon (1 teaspoon) Ground Black Pepper

- 1 teaspoon (1 teaspoon) Kosher Salt
- 1/2 teaspoon (0.5 teaspoon) Ground Nutmeg
- 1/4 cup (25 g) shredded Parmesan cheese

DIRECTIONS

1. Grease a 6 inch pan and set aside.
2. In the medium bowl, integrate spinach, onion, garlic, cream cheese dices, salt, pepper, and nutmeg. Pour into greased pan.
3. Set air fryer to 350°F for 10 mins. Open and stir the spinach to combine the cream cheese thru the spinach.
4. Sprinkle the Parmesan cheese on top. Set air fryer to 400°F for five mins or till the cheese has melted and browned.
5. To in addition lessen carbs, reduce down at the onions

18. Keto Jalapeno Poppers

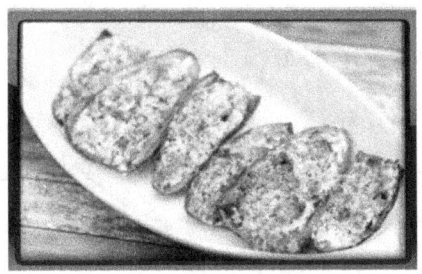

SERVING= 8 poppers

COOKING TIME = 20 minutes

Ingredients

- 4 jalapenos
- 3 ounces cream cheese, softened
- 1/2 cup shredded cheddar
- ½ teaspoon garlic powder
- ¼ teaspoon onion powder
- 4 slices bacon

DIRECTIONS

1. Slice jalapenos in 1/2 of length-wise. Carefully scrape out the seeds and membranes with a spoon and discard. See note.

2. 2. Add the cream cheese, cheddar, garlic powder, and onion powder to a small bowl and stir properly to combine.

3. 3. Spoon the cheese lightly among the jalapenos.

4. 4. Cut the bacon slices in 1/2 of and wrap every jalapeno with a 1/2 of slice of bacon.

Air Fryer Method:

1. Turn air fryer to 390 levels and allow warmth for two mins.

    2. Carefully upload the jalapenos to the basket of the air fryer in a unmarried layer
    with area among each. Work in batches in case your air fryer will now no
    longer match all eight halves at once.

    3. Air fry for 10 mins or till bacon is as crisp as you'd like.

19. AIR FRYER ROASTED BRUSSELS SPROUTS

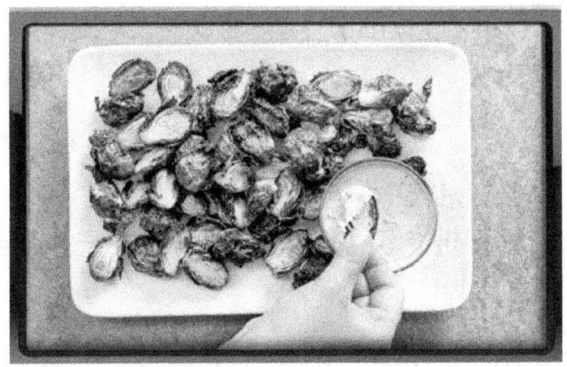

SERVING= 4

COOKING TIME = 18 minutes

Ingredients

- 1 lb. brussels sprouts (cleaned and trimmed)
- 1/2 tsp. dried thyme
- 1 tsp. dried parsley
- 1 tsp. garlic powder (Or 4 cloves, minced)
- 1/4 tsp. salt

- 2 tsp. Oil

DIRECTIONS

1. Place all elements in a medium to huge blending bowl and toss to coat the brussels sprouts evenly.
2. Pour them into the meals basket of the air fryer and near it up.
3. Set the warmth to 390 F. And the time to eight minutes. This putting roasts them well at the outdoor at the same time as leaving the insides a well cooked al dente.
4. Cool barely and serve.

20. AIR FRIED CAULIFLOWER RICE

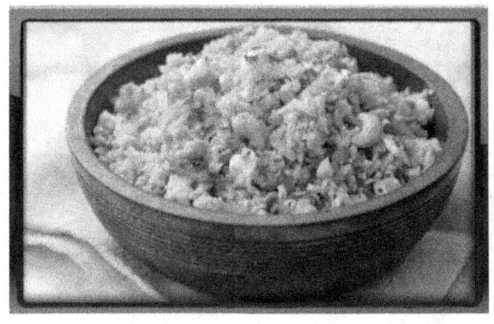

SERVING= 3

COOKING TIME = 30 minutes

INGREDIENTS

- 1/2 block firm or extra firm tofu
- 2 tablespoons reduced sodium soy sauce
- 1/2 cup diced onion
- 1 cup diced carrot - about 1 1/2 to 2 carrots
- 1 teaspoon turmeric
- 3 cups riced cauliflower - Cauliflower minced into pieces smaller than the size of a pea. You can do

this by hand with a box-style cheese crater, use your food processor to pulse into pieces, or buy pre-riced, bagged cauliflower.

- 2 tablespoons reduced sodium soy sauce
- 1 1/2 teaspoons toasted sesame oil - optional, but recommended
- 1 tablespoon rice vinegar
- 1 tablespoon minced ginger
- 1/2 cup finely chopped broccoli
- 2 cloves garlic - minced
- 1/2 cup frozen peas

DIRECTIONS

1. In a huge bowl, disintegrate the tofu (you're going for scrambled egg-length pieces, now no longer ricotta here), then toss with the relaxation of the Round 1 elements. Air fry at 370F for 10 mins, shaking once.
2. Meanwhile, toss collectively all the Round 2 elements in a huge bowl*.
3. When that first 10 mins of cooking are finished, upload all the Round 2 elements for

your air fryer, shake gently, and fry at 370 for 10 extra mins, shaking after five mins.

4. Riced cauliflower can range pretty a chunk in length, so in case you experience like yours doesn't appearance finished sufficient at this point, you may prepare dinner dinner for an extra 2-five mins at 370F. Just shake and take a look at in each short time till it's finished for your liking.

21.Keto Air Fryer Chickpeas

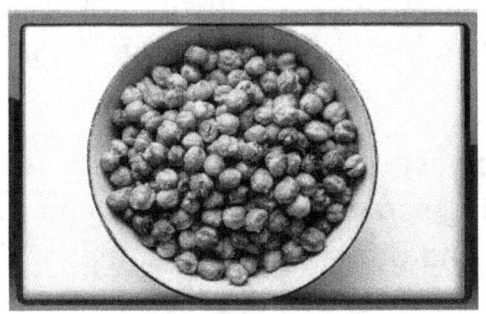

SERVING= 4

COOKING TIME = 22 minutes

INGREDIENTS

- 1 can Chickpeas
- 2 teaspoons Chili powder
- 2 teaspoons Cumin
- 2 teaspoons Grated lime zest
- 1 teaspoon Salt

DIRECTIONS

1. Add the Chickpeas to a medium-length bowl and blend with the chili powder, cumin, lime zest and salt.
2. Line the lowest of your air fryer with foil and spray with cooking spray. Place the chickpeas on pinnacle of the foil and prepare dinner dinner withinside the air fryer at 400F for 17 minutes.
3. Open the air fryer periodically and shake the chickpeas to make sure even cooking.
4. Cool absolutely and keep in an hermetic container.

22. Air Fryer Steak Bites and Mushrooms

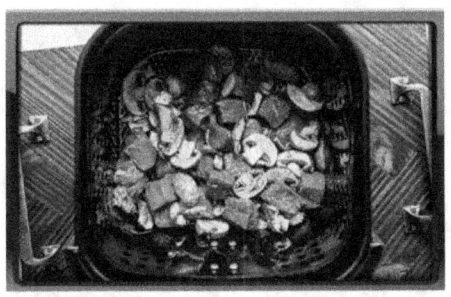

SERVING= 2

COOKING TIME = 1 Hour 20 minutes

INGREDIENTS

- 1 teaspoon kosher salt
- 1/2 teaspoon garlic powder
- 1/4 teaspoon black pepper
- 2 Tablespoons Worcestershire Sauce
- 2 Tablespoons avocado oil (Click here for my favorite brand on Amazon)
- 8 oz Baby Bella Mushrooms, sliced

- 1 pound Top Sirloin steak, cut into 1.5 inch cubes

DIRECTIONS

1. Combine all of your elements for the marinade right into a huge blending bowl.
2. Add your steak cubes and sliced mushrooms into your blending bowl with the marinade and toss to coat.
3. keep steak and mushrooms to marinate for 1 hour.
4. Pre-warmth your Air Fryer to 400F for five mins.
5. Make positive you spray the internal of your air fryer will cooking spray and pour your steak and mushrooms into the air fryer basket.
6. Cook the steak and mushrooms withinside the Air Fryer for five mins at 400F. Open the basket and shake the steak and mushrooms so that they prepare dinner dinner evenly. Continue to prepare dinner dinner for five mins more.
7. Check the steak the usage of an inner meat thermometer. If the steak has now no longer reached your favored doneness, keep to prepare dinner dinner in three minute durations till the thermometer positioned withinside the middle of one steak chunk reaches the favored temperature.

(Rare=125F, Medium-rare=130F, Medium=140F, Medium-well=150F, well-done=160F)

8. Serve

23. Tomato Basil Scallops

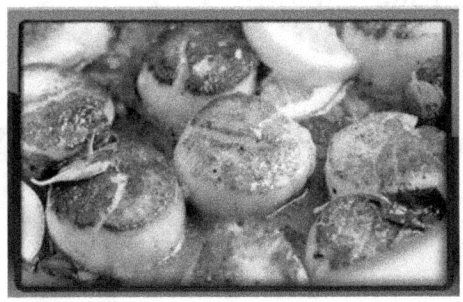

SERVING= 2

COOKING TIME = 15 minutes

Ingredients

- 3/4 cup (178.5 g) Heavy Whipping Cream
- 1 tablespoon (1 tablespoon) Tomato Paste
- 1 tablespoon (1 tablespoon) chopped fresh basil

- 1 teaspoon (1 teaspoon) Minced Garlic
- 1/2 teaspoon (0.5 teaspoon) Kosher Salt
- 1/2 teaspoon (0.5 teaspoon) Ground Black Pepper
- 1 12 oz (1 12 oz) Frozen Spinach, thawed and drained
- 8 (8) jumbo sea scallops
- Cooking Oil Spray
- additional salt and pepper to season scallops

DIRECTIONS

1. Spray a 7-inch heatproof pan, and vicinity the spinach in a good layer on the bottom.
2. Spray each aspects of the scallops with vegetable oil, sprinkle a touch greater salt and pepper on them, and vicinity scallops withinside the pan on pinnacle of the spinach.
3. In a small bowl, blend collectively the cream, tomato paste, basil, garlic, salt and pepper and pour over the spinach and scallops.
4. Set the airfryer to 350F for 10 mins till the scallops are cooked thru to an inner temperature of 135F

and the sauce is warm and bubbling. Serve immediately.

24. BEEF BULGOGI BURGERS

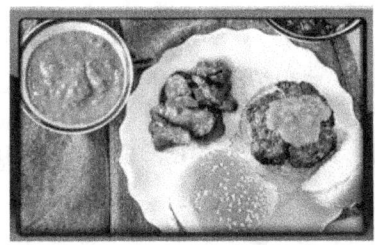

SERVING= 4

COOKING TIME = 25 minutes

INGREDIENTS

For the Bulgogi Burgers:

- 1 pound (453.59 g) Lean Ground Beef
- 2 tablespoon (2 tablespoon) gochujang
- 1 tablespoon (1 tablespoon) dark soy sauce
- 2 teaspoon (2 teaspoon) Minced Garlic
- 2 teaspoon (2 teaspoon) Minced Ginger
- 2 teaspoon (2 teaspoon) Sugar Or Other Sweetener Equivalent
- 1 tablespoon (1 tablespoon) Sesame Oil
- 1/4 cup (25 g) Chopped Green Scallions
- 1/2 tsp (0.5 tsp) Kosher Salt

For the Gochujang Mayonaisse

- 1/4 cup (56 g) Mayonnaise
- 1 tablespoon (1 tablespoon) gochujang
- 1 tablespoon (1 tablespoon) Sesame Oil
- 2 teaspoon (2 teaspoon) Sesame Seeds
- 1/4 cup (25 g) Chopped Green Scallions, chopped
- 4 (4) hamburger buns for serving

DIRECTIONS

1. In a massive bowl, blend floor beef, gochujang, soy sauce, garlic, ginger, sugar, sesame oil, chopped onions and salt and permit the combination to relaxation for half-hour or as much as 24 hours in a refrigerator.

2. Divide the beef into 4 quantities and shape spherical patties, with a moderate despair withinside the center to save you the burgers from puffing out right into a dome-form whilst cooking.

3. Set your air fryer to 360F for 10 mins and region the patties in a unmarried layer withinside the air fryer basket.

4. Make the Gochujang Mayonnaise: While the patties cook, blend collectively the mayonnaise, gochujang, sesame oil, sesame seeds and scallions.

5. Using a meat thermometer, make sure that the beef has reached an inner temperature of 160F and cast off to a serving tray.

6. Serve the patties with hamburger buns and the gochujang mayonnaise.

25. AIR FRYER ONION RINGS

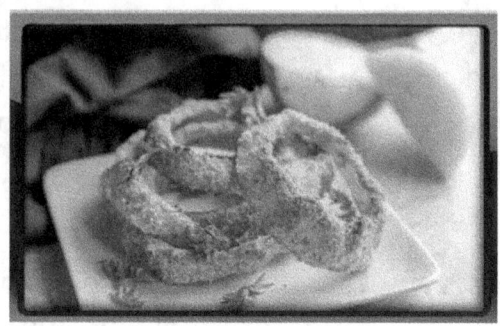

SERVING= 6

COOKING TIME = 30 minutes

INGREDIENTS

- 1 large Yellow Onion
- 2 eggs
- 3/4 cup Almond Flour
- 1/4 cup Ground Flax Seed
- 1/4 tsp Paprika
- 1/4 tsp Garlic Powder

- 1/2 tsp Salt
- 1/4 tsp Ground Black Pepper
- Spray Olive or Avocado Oil

DIRECTIONS

1. Spray avocado or vegetable oil spray on rock bottom of your air fryer basket and preheat to 400 degrees.
2. Take out 2 bowls. In one crack and scramble both eggs.
3. In the other, add almond flour, flax seed and spices and whisk together until fully combined.
4. Peel your onion and dig rings that are about 1/2 inch thick and pull apart each ring. Discard the within smaller rings or use them for something else. These might be made into onion rings if you do not mind the form .
5. Dip each onion ring into egg coating it evenly then press into flour mixture ensuring it's all evenly coated. Place each ring onto a plate until you've got a basket full before putting into air fryer.

6. Repeat above step until all onion rings are dredged and coated.

7. Next, spray your breaded onion rings with a lightweight coat of vegetable oil or avocado oil spray to make sure they get a pleasant crispy brown color.

8. Using tongs, place during a single layer into air fryer basket. don't over crowd the basket. Onion rings may have to be cooked in several batches.

9. Cook for 5-7 minutes and flip to cook another 5 minutes. Keep checking on them as they will burn quickly.

10. Once onion rings are cooked, serve immediately.

Part 2

Introduction

If you're following a ketogenic diet you don't need to worry about eating too much fat, but there are other benefits to frying with air instead of oil. Foods typically cook faster and there's less electricity used, compared to using a full-sized oven. Plus the amount of easy low-carb air fryer recipes to try is endless!
The appliance is perfect for cooking finger foods like keto appetizers, but it's also a great way to cook steaks, fish, chicken, and other proteins. Air frying is a fantastic way to cook chicken wings to achieve the perfect level of crispness as well.

Keep in mind, keto air fryer recipes often call for a small amount of oil. It's much less than you would use in deep frying, but you still get a nice, crispy coating and wonderful flavor with the air fryer. I find browning in the air fryer is more even than in the oven, especially if you occasionally toss or turn the food mid-cooking. The air fryer is much easier to clean than a deep fryer. Most parts simply go in the dishwasher.

With air fryers, there's really no limit to the amazing healthy recipes you can cook. If there are fried foods you're craving, an air fryer is a great way!

Chapter 1

Ketogenic Diets And Their Rapid Weight Loss Effects

Most weight-loss diets to varying degrees focus on either calorie reduction or the manipulation of the intake of one of the three essential macronutrients (proteins, fats, or carbohydrates) to achieve their weight loss effects.

Ketogenic diets are a group of "high-fat, moderate protein" or "high-protein moderate fat" but very low-carbohydrate diets. The term ketogenic basically refers to the increased production of ketone bodies occasioned by the elevated rate of lipolysis (fat break down). Ketones are the acidic by-products formed during the intermediate break down of "fat" into "fatty acids" by the liver.

The first sets of ketogenic diets were developed as far back as the early 1920s by the Johns Hopkins Pediatric Epilepsy Center to treat children seizures. The diets were designed to mimic the biochemical changes that occurred during periods of fasting, namely ketosis, acidosis, and dehydration. The diets involved the consumption of about 10-15 grams of carbohydrates per day, 1 gram of protein per kilogram body weight of the patient and the remaining calories derived from fats.

Today, promoters of ketogenic diets are of the view that carbohydrates especially the high glycemic index ones are the major reasons why people gain weight. Carbohydrate foods are generally metabolized to produce glucose, a form of simple sugar that is generally regarded as the preferred energy source for the body as it is faster burning energy. Although the body can break down muscle glycogen (a mixture of glucose and water) and fat to produce energy, it, however, prefers to get it from high glycemic index carbohydrates from diets.

Of the macronutrients, carbohydrates are therefore argued to be the major cause of weight gain. This is so because the increased intake of high glycemic index carbohydrate foods generally causes fluctuating blood sugar levels due to their fast absorption into the bloodstream and which more often than not leads to the overproduction of insulin. This is where the problem actually starts.

Insulin is a hormone that regulates blood glucose levels and therefore maintenance of the energy in/energy out equation of the body which rules body weight. Excess amounts of glucose in the bloodstream cause the excessive secretion of insulin which leads to the storage of the excess glucose in the body as either glycogen in liver and muscle cells or fat in fat cells.

One aim of ketogenic diets is, therefore, to reduce insulin production to its barest minimum by drastically reducing carbohydrate consumption while using fats and proteins to supplement the body's energy requirement.

Despite the ability of ketogenic diets to reduce insulin production, their main objective is ultimately aimed at inducing the state of ketosis. Ketosis can be regarded as a condition or state in which the rate of formation of ketones produced by the break down of "fat" into "fatty acids" by the liver is greater than the ability of tissues to oxidize them. Ketosis is a secondary state of the process of lipolysis (fat break down) and is a general side effect of low-carbohydrate diets. Ketogenic diets are therefore favorably disposed to the encouragement and promotion of ketosis.

Prolonged periods of starvation can easily induce ketosis but it can also be deliberately induced by making use of a low-calorie or low-carbohydrate diet through the ingestion of large amounts of either fats or proteins and drastically reduced carbohydrates. Therefore, high-fat and high-protein diets are the weight loss diets used to deliberately induce ketosis.

Essentially, ketosis is a very efficient form of energy production which does not involve the production of insulin as the body rather burns its fat deposits for energy. Consequently, the idea of reducing carbohydrate consumption does not only reduce insulin production but also practically forces the body to burn its fat deposit for energy, thereby making the use of ketogenic diets a very powerful way to achieve rapid weight loss.

Doing Aerobic Exercise With a Ketogenic Diet

Many prefer doing an exercise that is done with a combination of body movements; just like aerobic exercise with the cyclical ketogenic diet. It is not an easy way to do because it requires a lot of energy in performing it. This kind of exercise is not advisable to those who are on a restricted calorie diet specially when their energy is also affected. When doing an aerobic exercise you must have enough energy to accomplish it but how will you be able to do it if you are just eating a limited amount of food? Once an individual is on a diet he or she can only do limited activities. It can even make them easily get tired and become weak. This does not happen when you are on a ketogenic diet.

It doesn't mean that when you are already on a diet you will also become healthy. It is the most affected in your life because you are not eating enough food to give your body the nutrients that it needs. You may become slimmer but your health will be in great danger. The only thing you can do is to invest in dietary supplements that aside from losing weight it will also provide your body with the nutrients that it requires. There are a lot of products that promises this kind of benefits but most of it does not give your body the right amount of energy to do intense task. With the ketogenic diet, you will not just achieve the perfect body that you wish to have but you will also acquire a huge amount of energy that you can use to do other aerobic exercise.

Aerobic exercise with the ketogenic diet is the perfect combination that you can ever encounter since most of us want to have a physically fit and healthy body. With these two factors, you can achieve the body that you want and still have enough energy to do some exercise. Diet will always be useless if you will not do an exercise. Imagine yourself losing weight but not having a firm and fit body. This is what will most likely happen to you if you lack exercise when you are having your diet. You may reduce weight but your body structure will not be in perfect shape.

There are hundreds of companies that promote effective weight loss products as well as programs. To purchase the right one you must compare each of these and know its difference. You can set factors that you will follow base on what you want in a dietary product or program. With this process, it would be much easier for you to decide what brand you will purchase. However, in case you are haven't got any idea what to purchase, why not choose a ketogenic diet?. It has great benefits for anyone who will use it. With the combination of aerobic exercise and the ketogenic diet, you can be assured that you will not just be satisfied with the result but you will also be proud of it.

Chapter 2

5 Tips For Success on the Ketogenic Diet

Below are a few tips to maximize your success on a ketogenic diet.

1.) Drink alot of water.
While on a ketogenic diet, your body has a hard time retaining as much water as it needs, so staying properly hydrated is essential. Many experts recommend that men intake a minimum of 3 liters of beverages each day, while the figure for women is 2.2 liters daily. A good indicator of proper hydration is the color of your urine. If your urine is clear or light yellow, you're most likely properly hydrated. Keep a bottle of water with you everywhere you go!

2.) Don't forget the fat!
Simply put, our bodies need fuel to function. When we limit our carbohydrate intake, especially to levels that induce ketosis, our bodies need an alternate fuel source. Since protein is not an efficient source of energy, our bodies turn to fat. Any fat you eat while in ketosis is used for energy, making it very difficult to store fat while in ketosis. Choose healthy, unsaturated fats as often as possible: foods like avocados, olives, nuts, and seeds are ideal.

3.) Find your carb limit.

All of our bodies are different. Some dieters will need to adhere to a strict low-carbohydrate diet that entails consuming less than 20 grams per day of carbs. Other dieters will find that they can comfortably stay in ketosis while consuming 50, 75, or 100 grams of carbohydrates. The only way to know for sure is trial and error. Purchase Ketostix or any brand of ketone urinalysis strips and find out your carbohydrate limit. If you find that you have a bit of wiggle room, it will make sticking to your diet that much easier.

4.) Be smart about liquor.

One of the great aspects of the ketogenic diet is that you can drink liquor while on it without throwing your weight loss too far off course. You can drink unsweetened liquors like vodka, rum, tequila, gin, whiskey, scotch, cognac, and brandy, along with the occasional low-carb beer. Use low-carb mixers and drink plenty of water to stay hydrated, as hangovers are notoriously bad while in ketosis. And remember, calories still count, so don't go overboard. All things in moderation.

5.) Be patient.

While the ketogenic diet is known for rapid weight loss, especially in the early stages of the diet, weight loss is always a slow, time-consuming process. Don't freak out if the scale doesn't show weight loss, or shows slight weight increases, for a few days. Your weight varies day-to-day (and throughout the day) based upon a number of factors. Don't forget to use metrics like how your clothes fit or body measurements to see progress beyond what the scale shows.

The Cyclic Ketogenic Diet!

Athletes often use a cyclic ketogenic diet to maintain muscle mass and control fat. CKD's are based on a period in ketosis followed by a period of carbohydrate 'loading'. The theory behind CKD's is that breaking Ketosis every 5 to 10 days for 1-3 days of high carbohydrate intake will:
- Restore muscle glycogen
- Restore gym performance
- Rebuild any lost muscle (and hopefully add some new muscle)

A typical example of a cyclic ketogenic diet is as follows:

Six days of low carbohydrate consumption: Try to stay between 20 to 40 grams of carbohydrates per day, obtaining your nutrients from good sources of protein (meat, chicken, fish, eggs, etc.), fat (coconut oil, fish oil, avocado, butter, olive oil, etc.), green leaves (chard, lettuce, lavender, watercress, ammonia, asparagus, chicory, endive, spinach, arugula, parsley) and cruciferous vegetables (broccoli, cabbage, cauliflower, brussels sprouts, turnip, watercress, radish, and mustard).

A day of high carbohydrate consumption: For 24 hours, reverse the cycle and consume lots of carbohydrates and few fats, in order to replenish the glycogen supply and thus have the energy to continue practicing high-intensity physical exercises. Remember to get carbohydrates from good sources (fruits, vegetables, sweet potatoes, yams, cassava, etc.). Avoid wheat and sugar.

In a practical example, you can consume a lot of carbohydrates from 12 pm on Saturday until 12 pm on Sunday (taking two lunches) and staying the rest of the week on the low carbohydrate cycle.

If you want to get a good performance in your physical activity, try to put your workouts closer to that day of high carbohydrate consumption.

Challenge yourself to try the Cyclic ketogenic diet for at least a month to see the results!

Chapter 3

Category of Foods To Consume on Ketogenic Diet

Meat – Unprocessed meats are low carb and keto-friendly, and organic and grass-fed meat might be even healthier. But remember that keto is a higher-fat diet, not high in protein, so you don't need huge amounts of meat. Excess protein (over 2.0 g per kg of reference body weight; see this chart to determine your protein targets) can be converted to glucose, which could make it harder for some people to get into ketosis, especially when starting out and with high levels of insulin resistance.

Fish and seafood – These are all good, especially fatty fish like salmon. If you have concerns about mercury or other toxins, consider eating more of the smaller fish like sardines, mackerel, and herring. If you can find wild-caught fish, that's probably the best. Avoid breading, as it contains carbs.

Eggs – Eat them any way you want, e.g. boiled, fried in butter, scrambled or as omelets. Buying organic or pastured eggs might be the healthiest option, although we do not have scientific studies to prove better health.

Natural fat, high-fat sauces – Most of the calories on a keto diet should come from fat. You'll likely get much of it from natural sources like meat, fish, eggs, and other sources. But also use fat in cooking, like butter or coconut oil, and feel free to add plenty of olive oil to salads and vegetables. You can also eat delicious high-fat sauces, including Bearnaise sauce, garlic butter, and others (recipes).

Vegetables growing above ground. Fresh or frozen – either is fine. Choose vegetables growing above ground, especially leafy and green items. Favorites include cauliflower, cabbage, avocado, broccoli, and zucchini.

Vegetables are a tasty way to eat good fat on keto. Fry them in butter and pour plenty of olive oil on your salad. Some even think of vegetables as a fat-delivery system. They also add more variety, flavor, and color to your keto meals.

High-fat dairy – Butter is good, high-fat cheese is fine, and heavy cream is great for cooking.

Avoid drinking milk as the milk sugar quickly adds up (one glass = 15 grams of carbs), but you can use it sparingly in your coffee. What does "sparingly" mean? That depends on how many cups per day you drink! I recommend one cup with just a "splash," about a tablespoon max. But even better is to do away with the milk completely.

Nuts – Can be had in moderation, but be careful when using nuts as snacks, as it's very easy to eat far more than you need to feel satisfied. Also, be aware that cashews are relatively high carb, choose macadamia or pecan nuts instead.

Drinks –

Here is a list of what you can drink on a ketogenic diet:

Water – The #1 option. Have it flat, with ice, or sparkling. Sip it hot like a tea, or add natural flavoring like sliced cucumbers, lemons, or limes. If you experience headaches or symptoms of "keto flu", add a few shakes of salt to your water.10

Coffee – No sugar. A small amount of milk or cream is fine. For extra energy from fat, stir in butter and coconut oil for "Bulletproof coffee." Note, if weight loss stalls, cut back on the cream or fat in your coffee.

Tea – Whether black, green, Orange Pekoe, mint, or herbal — feel free to drink most teas. Don't add sugar.

Bone broth – Hydrating, satisfying, full of nutrients and electrolytes — and simple to make! — homemade bone broth can be a great beverage to sip on the keto diet. Stir in a pat of butter for some extra energy.

How an Air Fryer Complements a Low-Carb or Keto Diet

Cooking food for a low-carb or keto diet is challenging at times. Certain ingredients are restricted or off-limits which makes it difficult to create the foods you love. An air fryer can help make things easier if you're trying to follow a special eating plan.

Here are some ways an air fryer complements a low-carb diet:
- You can enjoy fried foods without the carbs
- It makes cooking at home faster and easier
- Versatile cooking options keep things interesting

Chapter 4: Delicious Air-Fryer Recipes

Breakfast Recipes

1. Eggs & Diary

Bacon & Egg Bite Cups

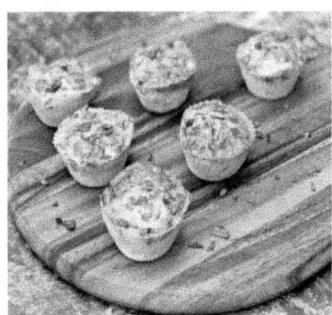

This low-carb and keto-friendly recipe shows how to cook eggs in the air fryer. This recipe uses silicone egg bite molds. Make these egg muffins whenever you want to meal prep omelets, quiche, or frittata!

Yield: 8

Total Time: 25 min

Ingredients

- 6 large eggs
- 2 tablespoons of heavy whipping cream or milk (any is fine)
- Salt and pepper to taste
- ¼ cup chopped green peppers
- ¼ cup chopped red peppers

- ¼ cup chopped onions
- ¼ cup chopped fresh spinach
- ½ cup shredded cheddar cheese
- ¼ cup shredded mozzarella cheese
- 3 slices of cooked and crumbled bacon

Instructions

Add the eggs to a large mixing bowl.

Add in the cream, salt and pepper to taste. Whisk to combine.

Sprinkle in the green peppers, red peppers, onions, spinach, cheeses, and bacon. I like to add only half of the ingredients here.

Whisk to combine.

I recommend you place the silicone molds in the air fryer before pouring in the egg mixture. This way you don't have to move the filled cups.

Pour the egg mixture into each of the silicone molds. If you have not used your molds yet, you may want to spray with cooking spray first to be sure.

Sprinkle in the remaining half of all the veggies.

Cook the egg bites cups for 12-15 minutes on 300 degrees. You can test the center of one with a toothpick. When the toothpick comes out clean, the eggs have set.

Recipe Notes

You can add half of the veggies to the eggs and then the other half to the top of the egg molds because it helps bring color to the outside of the eggs once baked. This isn't required.

If you want your bites to have melted cheese on top, save the cheese and add it at the end. When the egg bite cups have cooked for 10 minutes, open the air fryer and add the cheese. Cook until the eggs are set and the cheese has melted.

These egg bite cups are freezer friendly.

Nutrition

- Calories 119 kcal
- Total Fat 9g
- Carbohydrates 2g
- Protein 8g

Avocado With Eggs & Bacon

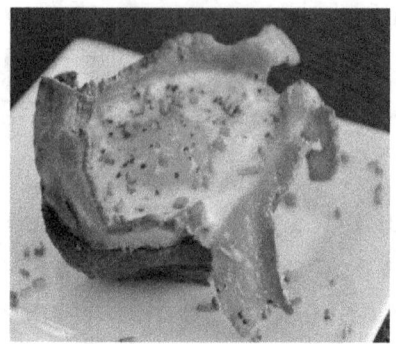

Total Time: 15 min

Servings: 2

Ingredients

- 1 ripe avocado
- 2 eggs
- 2 slices bacon, cooked and crumbled
- oil, for spraying
- 1 teaspoon cilantro or parsley, chopped

Directions

Cut avocado in half and remove seed. Scoop out just enough flesh to fit one egg without spilling. Drop one egg into each avocado half and sprinkle with crumbled bacon.

Place avocado halves in air fryer basket and spray with oil. Set the air fryer temperature to 350 degrees, and cook for 5 minutes, or until whites are set and yolks are runny. Sprinkle with cilantro or parsley and serve warm.

Nutrition

- Calories: 362.3 kcal
- Total Fat: 24.5g
- Net carbs: 2.6g
- Protein: 29.4g

Baked Egg Cups Spinach & Cheese

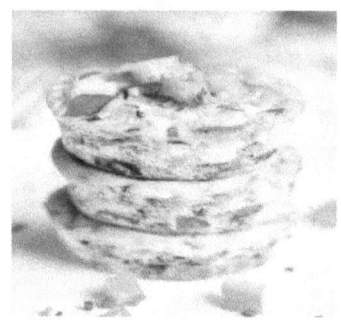

This recipe is written based on one egg, but you can cook as many in a batch that your air fryer will fit without squishing the baking vessels.

If cooking multiple cups at a time, it may take additional time. Or if you're making a 2 eggs in one jumbo sized muffin cup, add an additional 2-4 minutes.

Total Time: 15 mins

Serves: 4

Ingredients

- 1 large egg
- 1 tablespoon almond milk or half & half
- 1 tablespoon frozen spinach , thawed (or sautéed fresh spinach)
- 1-2 teaspoons grated cheese
- salt, to taste
- black pepper, to taste
- Cooking Spray, for muffin cups or ramekins

Directions

Spray inside of silicone muffin cups or ramekin with oil spray.

Add egg, milk, spinach and cheese into the muffin cup or ramekin.

Season with salt and pepper. Gently stir ingredients into egg whites without breaking the yolk.

Air Fry at 330°F for about 6-12 minutes (single egg cups usually take about 6 minutes - multiple or doubled up cups take as much as 12. As you add more egg cups, you will need to add more time.)

Cooking in a ceramic ramekin may take a little longer. If you want runny yolks, cook for less time. Keep checking the eggs after 5 minutes to ensure the egg is to your preferred texture.

Nutrition

- Calories 108 kcal
- Total Fat 9g
- Carbohydrates 2g
- Protein 8g

Bacon, Egg and Cheese Roll-Ups

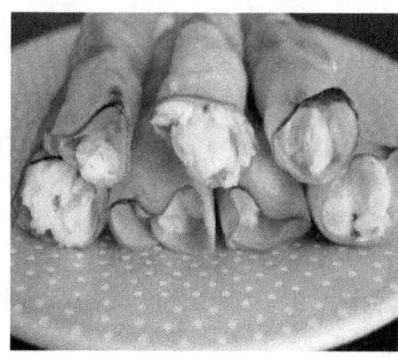

This Low Carb Bacon, Egg, and Cheese Roll-Ups are the ultimate keto breakfast. Scrambled eggs and cheese are rolled up in bacon slices and then air fried until the bacon gets crispy.

Total Time: 30 minutes

Servings: 2

Ingredients

- 2 tablespoons butter
- 1/2 cup chopped onion
- 1/2 cup chopped green bell pepper
- 4 large eggs
- salt and pepper
- 6 slices sugar-free bacon
- 2/3 cup shredded cheddar cheese
- 1/3 cup hot salsa

Instructions

Melt butter in a medium nonstick skillet over medium heat. Add onion and peppers and cook 3 minutes to soften.

Whisk eggs and season with salt and pepper. Add to pan with onion and peppers and scramble. Remove pan from the heat while eggs are still a little undercooked. You need them cooked enough to hold theie form, but they will finish cooking in the air fryer.

Place 3 slices of bacon side by side. Place half of the scrambled egg mixture towards the end nearest you.

Place half the cheddar on top of the eggs.

Roll bacon around eggs and secure with a toothpick. Repeat with remaining bacon and eggs.

Place in air fryer basket. Set temperature to 350 degrees for 15 minutes. Flip over half-way through.

Serve with salsa for dipping.

Nutrition

- Calories 680 kcal
- Fat 61g
- Carbohydrates 9.1g
- Protein 33g

Scrambled Eggs

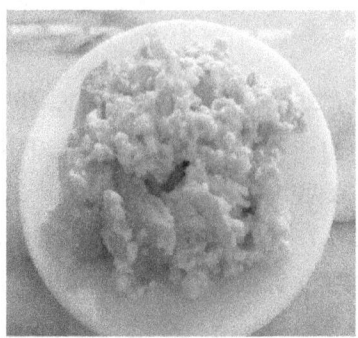

An easy way to make scrambled eggs inside your air fryer to perfection.

Total Time: 12 Min

Serves: 2

Ingredients

- 1/3 tablespoon unsalted butter
- 2 eggs
- 2 tablespoons almond milk
- salt and pepper to taste
- 1/8 cup cheddar cheese

Instructions

Place butter in an air fryer-safe pan and place inside the air fryer.

Cook at 300 degrees until butter is melted, about 2 minutes.

Whisk together the eggs and milk, then add salt and pepper to taste.

Cook on 300 degrees for 3 minutes, then push eggs to the inside of the pan to stir them around.

Cook for 2 more minutes then add cheddar cheese, stirring the eggs again.

Cook 2 more minutes.

Remove pan from air fryer and enjoy immediately.

Nutrition

- Calories: 126 kcal
- Total Fat: 9g
- Net Carbohydrates: 1g
- Protein: 9g

Scotch Eggs

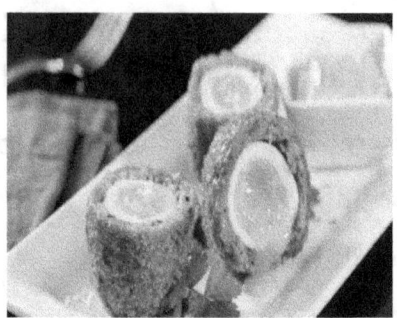

Scotch eggs are the perfect breakfast and brunch dish. It's always a great conversation piece when everyone sees the boiled egg stuffed in sausage. Use whatever your favorite sausage might be: Sweet Italian, Breakfast Sausage, Chicken Apple, etc. Don't forget the swipe of mustard and hot sauce.

Total Time: 30 mins

Servings: 6

Ingredients

- 1 pound uncooked bulk sausage
- 5-6 hard boiled eggs
- 1-2 raw eggs , beaten
- 1 cup coating choice (crushed pork rinds, almond flour, coconut flour or preferred coating *see notes below)
- Mustard and/or hot sauce oil spray, for coating

Directions

Peel hard boiled eggs. Divide the sausage into 5 or 6 equal parts, depending on how thick you want the sausage to wrap around the egg.

Flatten each portion into a thin patty about 4" wide. Lay boiled egg in center and wrap sausage around the whole egg. Repeat for all eggs.

Dip sausage-wrapped egg in beaten raw egg, then in breading. Spray outside of coated egg evenly with oil.

Air Fry at 400°F for 12-16 minutes, turn halfway through cooking. The thicker the sausage layer, the longer it takes to cook.

Cut in half and serve with mustard swipe on top of yolk. Add hot sauce, too, if you want. Enjoy!!!

Recipe Notes

You can add additional flavor to your sausage by mixing it with some Worcestershire, fresh parsley and other spices. If not, simple bulk sausage still tastes great!

Coating Choice: If you don't mind a few more carbs, bread crumbs, panko flakes, or crushed crackers work great as breading choices too. For fewer calories, you can omit the coatings (beaten egg & breading). The sausage-only outside is great, too, but make sure to spray outside of sausage with oil.

Nutrition

- Calories 323 kcal

- Fat 26g
- Carbohydrates 1g
- Protein 20g

Baked Potted Egg

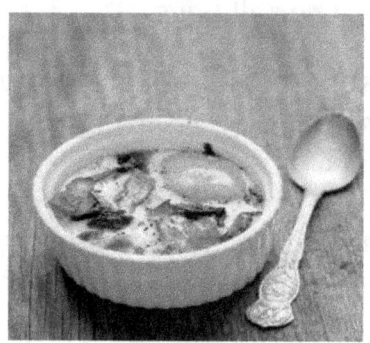

Total Time: 17 Minutes

Serves: 3

Ingredients

- 3 eggs
- 6 slices smoked streaky bacon, diced
- 2 cups baby spinach, washed
- ⅓ cup heavy cream
- 3 tablespoons Parmesan cheese, grated
- Salt & pepper, to taste

Directions

Select preheat on the cosori air fryer, adjust to 350°f, and press start/pause.

Spray three 3-inch ramekins with nonstick cooking spray.

Add 1 egg to each greased ramekin.

Cook the bacon in a pan until crispy, about 5 minutes.

Add the spinach and cook until wilted, about 2 minutes.

Mix in the heavy cream and Parmesan cheese. Cook for 2 to 3 minutes.

Pour the cream mixture on top of the eggs.

Place the ramekins into the preheated air fryer and cook for 4 minutes at 350°F, until the egg white is fully set.

Season to taste with salt and pepper.

This tasty egg pot is rich in protein, helping you feel fuller for longer.

Nutrition

- 195 kcal
- 18g protein
- 1g Sugar
- 8g fat

2. Beef Recipe

Meatloaf Sliders

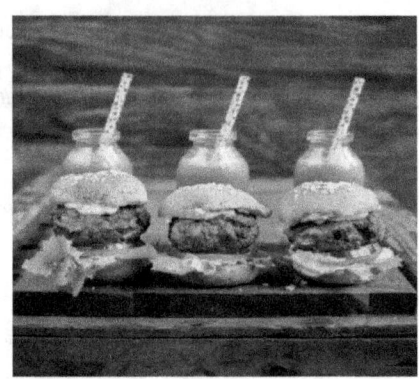

Total Time: 20 min

Yield: 8

Ingredients

- 1 lb ground beef
- 2 eggs, beaten
- ¼ cup onion, finely chopped
- 1 clove garlic, minced
- ½ cup blanched almond flour, extra is fine
- ¼ cup coconut flour
- ¼ cup ketchup
- ½ tsp sea salt
- ½ tsp black pepper
- 1 Tbsp Worcestershire Sauce
- 1 tsp Italian Seasoning
- ½ tsp Tarragon, dried

Instructions

In a large mixing bowl, combine all the ingredients and mix well. Make patties that are

about 2" in diameter and about 1" thick. If you want to make thicker or thinner patties,

make sure all of them are similar in size, so they cook properly at the same time. Place the patties on a platter and refrigerate for 10 minutes for the flour to absorb the wet ingredients and the patties to become firm.

Preheat the air fryer to 360°F.

Place as many patties you can fit in the basket and close. Set the timer for 10 minutes.

Check the patties half way. When the timer goes off, take them out to a serving platter and cover until all the patties are cooked.

Nutrition

- Calories: 228 kcal
- Fats: 9g
- Carbohydrates: 4g
- Protein: 13g

3. Sea Foods

Coconut Shrimp

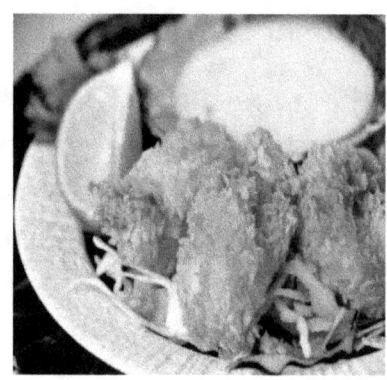

This keto coconut shrimp is crispy, full of flavor, and low carb. You can use ground pork rinds for the coating to make it keto approved, and pair it with a sriracha dipping sauce. The coconut shrimp recipe can be made in the air fryer or deep fryer.

Total Time: 21 min

Servings: 3

Ingredients

For The Shrimp:

- 1 pound shrimp peeled & cleaned
- ¾ cup all-purpose flour
- 1 teaspoon each onion & garlic powder
- 2 eggs lightly beaten

- ½ cup each panko breadcrumbs & unsweetened shredded coconut flakes
- Kosher salt & fresh pepper
- Avocado or grapeseed oil
- ½ cup full fat mayonnaise
- Zest & juice of half a lime
- 1 clove garlic, finely grated
- 2-3 tablespoons sriracha or hot sauce

For The Keto Coconut Shrimp:

- ¾ cup coconut flour
- 1 teaspoon each onion & garlic powder
- 2 eggs lightly beaten
- ½ cup each pork rind crumbs & unsweetened shredded coconut flakes
- Kosher salt & fresh pepper
- Avocado or grapeseed oil

Instructions

For the keto coconut shrimp, prepare the dredge station by adding the coconut flour, onion & garlic powder, ½ teaspoon salt, and a few cracks of pepper to a shallow dish, mix well. Add the eggs to a small dish/bowl and lightly whisk. Add the pork rinds to a zip-top bag and use a rolling pin to bash them into breadcrumbs the size of panko. Add them to a dish along with the coconut flakes, ¼ teaspoon salt, few cracks of pepper, and mix well.

Season the shrimp with a little pinch of salt on bot sides then dredge in the coconut flour shake off any excess, dredge in the eggs, shake off any excess, dredge in the pork rind and coconut flakes and make sure the shrimp is well covered. Move shrimp to a wire rack set over a sheet tray. Repeat the process with the remaining shrimp.

For the regular version of the coconut shrimp, follow the same exact steps but you use all-purpose flour instead of coconut, and panko breadcrumbs instead of pork rinds.

Pour 2 inches of oil into a frying pan and bring the temperature to 340-350 F. While the oil is coming to temperature, it's ok that the shrimp sit at room temperature so the coating can firm up. Fry the shrimp in batches, for 2-3 minutes on each side, or until golden brown. Remove shrimp and place on a clean wire rack and fry the next batch.

Make the sriracha dipping sauce by combining all the ingredients in a small bowl and whisking well. Check for seasoning, you may need more sriracha if you like it spicy.

If using an air fryer to make the coconut shrimp, spray the basket with non-stick and fry for 8 minutes at 390 F, flipping the shrimp half way.

Nutrition

- 75 kcal
- 0.9 net carbs
- 4 grams of fat

- 3.2 grams of protein

Fish Sticks

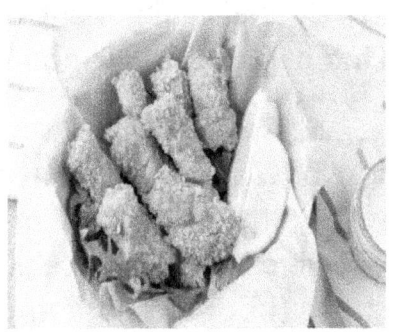

Crispy breaded keto fish sticks! This air fryer fish recipe is so simple and a total family pleaser.

Total Time: 20 mins

Servings: 4

Ingredients

- 1 lb white fish such as cod
- 1/4 cup mayonnaise
- 2 tbsp Dijon mustard
- 2 tbsp water
- 1 1/2 cups pork rind panko (such as Pork King Good)
- 3/4 tsp cajun seasoning
- Salt and pepper to taste

Instructions

Spray the air fryer rack with non-stick cooking spray (You can use avocado oil spray).

Pat the fish dry and cut into sticks about 1 inch by 2 inches wide (how you are able to cut it will depend a little on what kind of fish you by and how thick and wide it is).

In a small shallow bowl, whisk together the mayo, mustard, and water. In another shallow bowl, whisk together the pork rinds and Cajun seasoning. Add salt and pepper to taste (both the pork rinds and seasoning could have a fair bit of salt so dip a finger in to taste how salty it is).

Working with one piece of fish at a time, dip into the mayo mixture to coat and then tap off the excess. Dip into the pork rind mixture and toss to coat. Place on the air fryer rack.

Set to Air Fry at 400F and bake 5 minutes, the flip the fish sticks with tongs and bake another 5 minutes. Serve immediately.

Nutrition

- Calories 263 kcal
- Fat 16g
- Carbohydrates 1g
- Protein 26.4g

Crab Cakes

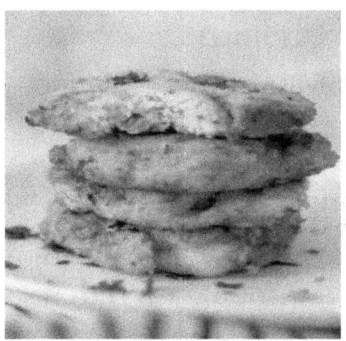

Making homemade Crab Cakes is easier when you use your air fryer! They turn out perfectly. Top them with an easy lemon and Old Bay aioli for a real treat!

Total Time: 20 minutes

Servings: 5

Ingredients

- 18 oz Canned Lump Crab Meat drained
- 2 Large Eggs
- 2 1/2 tbsp Mayonnaise
- 1 1/2 tbsp Dijon Mustard
- 1 tsp Old Bay Seasoning
- 1 tbsp Dried Celery
- 2 tsp Dried Parsley
- 1/4 cup Almond Flour
- 1/2 tsp Salt

Easy Lemon and Old Bay Aioli:

- 1/4 cup Mayonnaise
- 1/2 tsp Old Bay Seasoning
- 2-3 tsp Lemon Juice
- 1 tsp Dijon Mustard

Instructions

Combine all the ingredients for crab cakes in a large bowl. Gently fold everything together being careful not to break up the crab meat too much.

Line the basket or tray of your air fryer with aluminum foil and grease with oil or nonstick spray.

NOTE: If your air fryer has more then one rack, only use one at a time for best results.

Scoop 1/4 cup of the crab mixture onto the prepared aluminum foil, and form into a circle about 1/2 inch thick. You should be able to make about 10 crab cakes.

Cook the crab cakes at 320 degrees for 10 minutes, flipping after 5 minutes.

To prepare the aioli, simply combine all ingredients in a small bowl.

Serve the crab cakes topped with the aioli if desired.

Nutrition

- Calories: 194 kcal
- Carbohydrates: 1g
- Protein: 22g
- Fat: 10g

Tomato Mayonnaise Shrimp

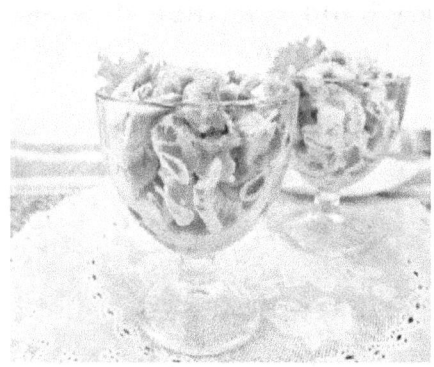

Tomato Mayonnaise Shrimp is so much more sophisticated-tasting than it sounds! Combine some spice with creamy ingredients to make an amazing appetizer.

Total Time: 13 minutes

Servings: 4

Ingredients

- 1 pound large 21-25 count peeled, tail-on shrimp
- 3 tablespoons mayonnaise
- 1 tablespoon Ketchup
- 1 tablespoon Minced Garlic
- 1 teaspoon Sriracha Sauce
- 1/2 teaspoon Smoked Paprika
- 1/2 teaspoon Salt

For Finishing

- 1/2 cup Green Onions

Instructions

In a medium bowl, mix together mayo, ketchup, garlic, sriracha, paprika, and salt.

Add the shrimp and toss to coat with the sauce.

Spray the airfryer basket. Place the shrimp into the greased basket.

Set airfryer to 325F for 8 minutes or until shrimp are cooked, tossing half way through and spraying with oil again.

Sprinkle chopped onions before serving.

Nutrition

- Calories: 196 kcal
- Carbohydrates: 2g
- Protein: 23g
- Fat: 9g

4. Vegetables

Delicious Roasted Veggies

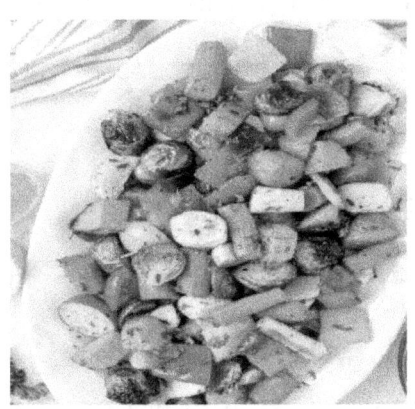

Total Time: 30 min

Servings: 4

Ingredients

- 1/2 cup diced zucchini
- 1/2 cup diced summer squash
- 1/2 cup diced mushrooms
- 1/2 cup diced cauliflower
- 1/2 cup diced asparagus
- 1/2 cup diced sweet red pepper
- 2 teaspoons vegetable oil
- 1/4 teaspoon salt
- 1/4 teaspoon ground black pepper
- 1/4 teaspoon desired seasoning (ideas below), or more to taste

Directions

Preheat the air fryer to 360 degrees F (180 degrees C).

Add vegetables, oil, salt, pepper, and desired seasoning to a bowl. Toss to coat; arrange in fryer basket.

Cook vegetables for 10 minutes, stirring after 5 minutes.

4 seasoning ideas

1. Italian seasoning
2. Herbes de Provence
3. Smoked paprika
4. Gremolata: 1/2 cup chopped fresh parsley, 2 teaspoons lemon zest, and 2 cloves minced garlic

Nutrition Facts

Per Serving:

- 37 kcal
- 2.4g fat
- 0.9g carbohydrates
- 1.4g protein

Zucchini Pizza Boats

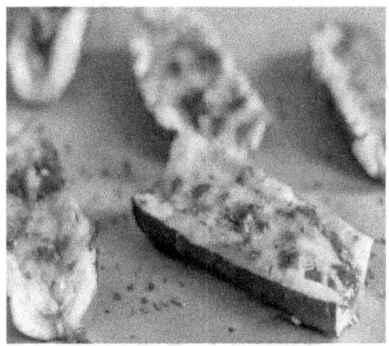

Make easy Zucchini Pizza Boats in the Air Fryer. These are low-carb and keto-friendly!

Total Time: 13 min

Yield: 8

Ingredients

- 2 Zucchini (More if they are small)
- 1/4 Cup Pizza Sauce
- Mini Pepperoni
- Shredded Mozzarella Cheese
- Olive oil spray

Instructions

Cut the zucchini in half if they are long and then again lengthwise.

Scoop the middle portion out with a spoon.

Spray the zucchini lightly with olive oil spray.

Add in the pizza sauce, top with pepperoni and cheese.

Place them in the air fryer basket.

Coat with an even coat of olive oil spray.

Air fry at 350 degrees for 8 minutes.

Add an additional 2 minutes if needed to crisp the cheese.

Repeat if necessary for the additional zucchini.

Nutrition

- Calories: 61 kcal
- Total Fat: 4g
- Carbs: 3g
- Protein: 2.4g

Sausage Balls

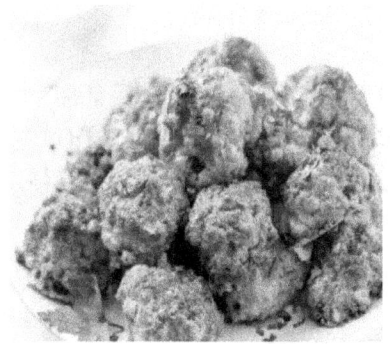

This recipe is one of a kind you can make all year long. It freezes beautifully and is perfect to have on hand in the event of unexpected guests. You won't believe how flavor-packed these little nibbles are.

Total Time: 26 mins

Servings: 16

Ingredients

- 1 3/4 cups almond flour
- 1 tablespoon baking powder
- 1/2 teaspoon sea salt
- 1/4 teaspoon ground black pepper
- 1/4 teaspoon cayenne pepper
- 1 pound sausage crumbled
- 8 ounces grated cheddar cheese
- 8 ounces cream cheese softened and cut into chunks

Instructions

In a large mixing bowl, combine almond flour, baking powder, salt, ground black pepper, and cayenne pepper.

Add sausage, cheddar cheese, and cream cheese. Stir to combine and then use clean hands to mix until all of the ingredients are well incorporated.

Form into balls about 1 1/2 inches.

Place in a single layer in your air fryer and spray. Set your air fryer to 350 degrees. Cook for 7 minutes and flip.

Respray and cook for 7 minutes longer, until lightly golden brown.

Nutrition

- Calories: 262 kcal
- Carbohydrates: 4g
- Protein: 11g
- Fat: 23g

Cauliflower With Buffalo Sauce

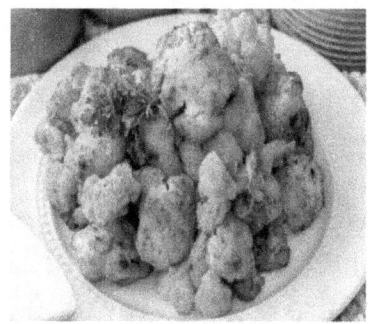

Enjoy these Vegetarian Cauliflower Buffalo Wings in the air fryer. These wings are delicious, low carb and gluten-free.

Total Time: 20 minutes

Servings 4

Ingredients

- 1 head cauliflower cut into small bites
- cooking oil spray
- 1/2 cup buffalo sauce (check recipe below)
- 1 tablespoon butter melted
- salt and pepper to taste

Instructions

Spray the air fryer basket with cooking oil.

Add the melted butter, buffalo sauce, and salt and pepper to taste to a bowl. Stir to combine.

Add the cauliflower bites to the air fryer. Spray with cooking oil. Cook for 7 minutes on 400 degrees.

Open the air fryer and place the cauliflower in a large mixing bowl. Drizzle the butter and buffalo mixture throughout. Stir.

Add the cauliflower back to the air fryer. Cook for an additional 7-8 minutes on 400 degrees until the cauliflower wings are crisp. Every air fryer brand is different. Be sure to use your personal judgment to assist with optimal cook time.

Remove the cauliflower from the air fryer. Serve with homemade Keto Ranch Dressing.

Recipe Notes: How to Make Buffalo Sauce

Total Time: 15 minutes

Servings: 16

Ingredients

- 1 1/3 cup Frank's red hot sauce
- 1 cup unsalted butter (2 sticks)
- 3 tablespoons white vinegar
- 1/2 teaspoon Worcestershire sauce
- 1/2 teaspoon cayenne pepper
- 1/4 teaspoon garlic powder
- 1/4 teaspoon paprika
- salt to taste

Instructions

In a saucepan over medium heat, combine the hot sauce, butter, vinegar, Worcestershire sauce, pepper, garlic powder and paprika.

Whisk often as the butter melts and allow the mixture to come to a simmer.

Once the sauce comes to a simmer, remove the pan from the heat.

Allow the sauce to cool slightly. Add a dash or two of salt, to taste.

The sauce will thicken as it cools. Whisk the sauce before serving over wings.

Refrigerate any leftovers. As you refrigerate the mixture, some of the butter may separate and harden. Simply reheat the mixture on the stovetop or microwave to make the sauce smooth again.

This mixture makes enough to cover 5 pounds of wings and have extra.

Nutrition

- Calories: 120 kcal
- Carbs: 2g
- Protein: 15g
- Fats: 10g

Spinach & Artichoke Dip

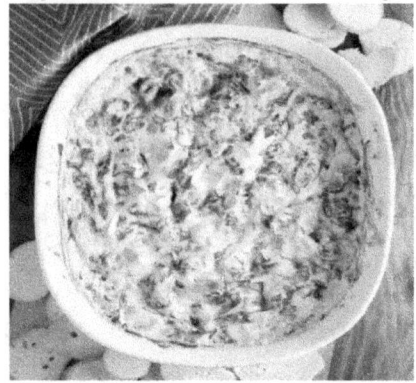

This Air Fryer Spinach and Artichoke Dip Recipe is just the appetizer you need for holiday feasts, parties and game day tables. Yes, you can make dip right in your air fryer!

Total time: 15 minutes

Serves: 2

Ingredients

- 3 Cups Fresh Baby Spinach - chopped
- 1 Tablespoon Oil
- 8 ounces Cream Cheese - softened
- 1/4 Cup Sour Cream
- 1/4 Cup Mayonnaise
- 1-2 Garlic Cloves - peeled, grated
- 1/2 teaspoon Garlic Powder
- 1/2 teaspoon Dried Italian Seasoning
- 1/4 teaspoon Onion Powder
- Salt/Pepper - to taste

- 1/2 Cup Chopped Marinated Artichoke Hearts
- 2 Cups Shredded Monterey Jack Cheese (or mozzarella) - divided
- Fresh Chopped Parsley

Instructions

Heat oil in a sauté pan over medium heat. Add fresh spinach and cook until spinach is wilted. (approx 5 minutes) Allow spinach to cool 5-10 minutes then transfer to paper towels or a fine mesh strainer. Remove as much liquid as possible.

In large bowl combine cream cheese, sour cream, mayo, garlic, garlic powder, Italian season, onion powder, salt and pepper. Use a hand mixer to produce a smooth, fluffy base.

Stir in wilted spinach, chopped artichokes and 1 cup shredded cheese. Transfer mixture to a 1 quart oven safe dish.

Place dip dish directly onto air fryer basket. Air fry at 375ºF for 5 minutes.

Top with 1 more cup of shredded cheese.

Air fry at 375ºF for 4-6 more minutes or until top is browned and bubbly.

Sprinkle with fresh chopped parsley and serve hot.

Nutrition

- Calories: 297 kcal

- Total Fat: 27g
- Carbs: 4g
- Protein: 10g

Creamed Spinach

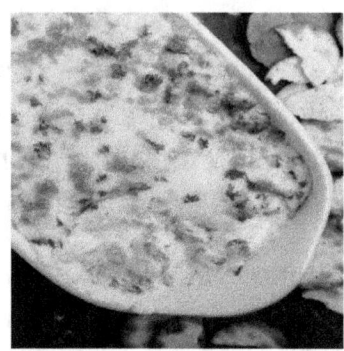

This recipe is creamy, low carb and ready in just 25 min in your air fryer.

Total Time: 25 minutes

Servings: 2

Ingredients

- 1 10 ounce package frozen spinach, thawed
- 1/2 cup onions, chopped
- 2 teaspoons Minced Garlic
- 4 ounces Cream Cheese, diced
- 1 teaspoon Ground Black Pepper
- 1 teaspoon Salt
- 1/2 teaspoon Ground Nutmeg
- 1/4 cup shredded Parmesan cheese

Instructions

Grease a 6 inch pan and set aside.

In the medium bowl, combine spinach, onion, garlic, cream cheese dices, salt, pepper, and nutmeg. Pour into greased pan.

Set air fryer to 350°F for 10 minutes. Open and stir the spinach to mix the cream cheese through the spinach.

Sprinkle the Parmesan cheese on top. Set air fryer to 400°F for 5 minutes or until the cheese has melted and browned.

To further reduce carbs, cut down on the onions

Nutrition

- Calories: 273 kcal
- Carbohydrates: 8g
- Protein: 8g
- Fat: 23g

Breakfast Casserole

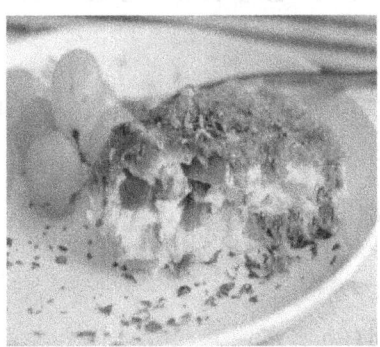

Very delcious casserole in an Air Fryer!

Total Time: 25 min

Yield: 8

Ingredients

- 1 lb Ground Sausage
- 1/4 Cup Diced White Onion
- 1 Diced Green Bell Pepper
- 8 Whole Eggs, Beaten
- 1/2 Cup Shredded Colby Jack Cheese
- 1 Tsp Fennel Seed
- 1/2 Tsp Garlic Salt

Instructions

If you are using the Ninja Foodi, use the saute function to brown the sausage in the pot of the foodi. If you are using an air fryer, you can use a skillet to do this.

Add in the onion and pepper and cook along with the ground sausage until the veggies are soft and the sausage is cooked.

Using the 8.75 inch pan or the Air Fryer pan, spray it with non-stick cooking spray.

Place the ground sausage mixture on the bottom of the pan.

Top evenly with cheese.

Pour the beaten eggs evenly over the cheese and sausage.

Add fennel seed and garlic salt evenly over the eggs.

Place the rack in the low position in the Ninja Foodi, and then place the pan on top.

Set to Air Crisp for 15 minutes at 390 degrees.

If you are using an air fryer, place the dish directly into the basket of the air fryer and cook for 15 minutes at 390 degrees.

Carefully remove and serve.

Nutrition

- Calories: 282 kcal
- Total Fat: 23g
- Sugar: 2g
- Protein: 15g

Stuffed Peppers

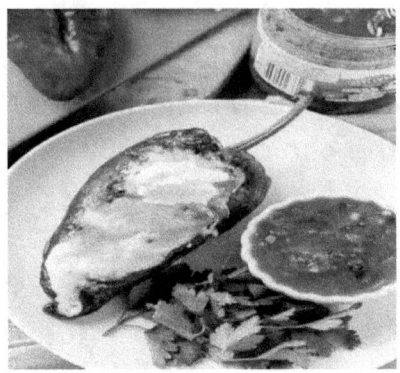

Air fryer breakfast stuffed peppers are the perfect low carb start to the day! A tender bell pepper filled with eggs you can eat and enjoy!

Total Time: 18 minutes

Servings: 2

Ingredients

- 1 bell pepper halved, middle seeds removed
- 4 eggs
- 1 tsp olive oil
- 1 pinch salt and pepper

Instructions

Cut bell peppers in half lengthwise and remove seeds and middle leaving the edges in tact like bowls.

Use your finger to rub a bit of olive oil just on the exposed edges (where it was cut).

Crack two eggs into each bell pepper half. Sprinkle with desired spices.

Set them on a trivet inside your Ninja Foodi or directly inside your other brand of air fryer.

Close the lid on your air fryer.

Turn machine on, press air crisper button at 390 degrees for 13 minutes.

Alternatively if you'd rather have your bell pepper and egg less brown on the outside add just one egg to your pepper and set air fryer to 330 degrees for 15 minutes (for an over hard egg consistency).

NUTRITION

- Calories 164 kcal
- Fat 10g
- Sugar 2g
- Protein 11g

Breakfast Frittata

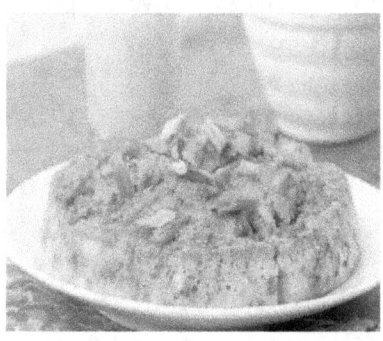

This Air Fryer Frittata is a quick, easy and protein-packed way to start your day!

Total Time: 25 min

Servings: 4

Ingredients

- 4 eggs
- 3 tablespoons heavy cream double cream
- 4 tablespoons grated cheddar cheese
- 4 mushrooms sliced
- 3 grape tomatoes cherry tomatoes, halved
- 4 tablespoons chopped spinach
- 2 tablespoons fresh chopped herbs of choice
- 1 green onion sliced
- salt to taste

Instructions

Preheat the air fryer to 350 F / 180 C.

Line a deep 7-inch baking pan with parchment paper, then oil the pan and set it aside.

In a bowl, whisk together the eggs and cream.

Add the rest of the ingredients to the bowl, and stir to combine.

Pour the breakfast frittata mixture into the baking pan and place inside the air fryer basket.

Cook for 12-16 minutes, or until eggs are set. To check, insert a toothpick in the center of the air fryer frittata. The eggs are set if it comes out clean.

Cooking Tips

As the eggs can stick to the pan, lining it with parchment and then oiling it is important.

Feel free to vary the veggies in this recipe to suit your taste. Just make sure to stick with quick cooking veggies.

This breakfast frittata is a great way to use up any leftover meat you might have. Toss in some diced ham, shredded chicken, or crumbled bacon.

Chef's Tip: if you want to avoid having your breakfast frittata get overly brown on top, cover the pan with foil before cooking and then remove it when halfway done.

Nutrition

- Calories: 147 kcal
- Carbohydrates: 3g
- Protein: 9g
- Fat: 11g

5. Chicken Recipes

Crispy Chicken Wings

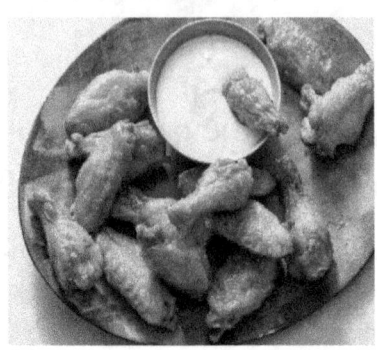

A step-by-step guide for how to cook chicken wings in an air fryer!

Total Time: 40 minutes

Serves: 8

Ingredients

- 2 lb Chicken wings (flats and drumettes, either fresh or thawed from frozen)
- 1 tbsp Gluten-free baking powder
- 3/4 tsp Sea salt
- 1/4 tsp Black pepper

Instructions

In a large bowl, toss the wings with baking powder, sea salt and black pepper.

Grease 2 racks for the air fryer oven. (If your air fryer only has a basket, grease that instead.)

Place the wings onto the greased racks, or place only enough wings into the basket to be in a single layer. (You may need to cook in 2 batches if using a basket.)

Place the racks or basket into the air fryer and cook for 15 minutes at 250 degrees.

Flip the wings over and switch the trays, so that the top is on the bottom and vice versa. Increase temperature to 430 degrees (or the highest your air fryer goes). Air fry for about 15 to 20 minutes, until chicken wings are done and crispy.

Nutrition

- Calories 275 kcal
- Fat 19g
- Protein 22g
- Total Carbs 1g

Tandoori Chicken Recipe

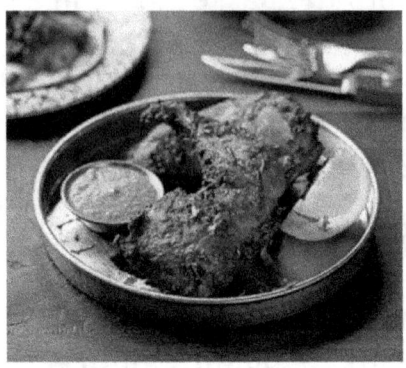

Make this Tandoori Chicken Recipe in your air fryer with a yogurt-based marinade. It's a flavor-packed, low carb chicken recipe that is super easy to make!

Total Time: 45 minutes

Servings: 4

Ingredients

- 1 pound chicken tenders, each cut in half
- ¼ cup Greek Yogurt
- 1 tablespoon minced ginger
- 1 tablespoon Minced Garlic
- ¼ cup Cilantro, or sub parsley
- 1 teaspoon Salt
- 1 teaspoon Cayenne
- 1 teaspoon Turmeric
- 1 teaspoon Garam Marsala
- 1 teaspoon (1 teaspoon) Smoked Paprika, to add a smoky flavor to the chicken, and color

For Finishing

- 1 tablespoon oil, or ghee for basting
- 2 teaspoons lemon juice, for finishing
- 2 tablespoons chopped cilantro, for garnishing

Instructions

In a glass bowl, mix all ingredients except the basting oil, lemon juice and 2 tablespoons of cilantro. Marinate for 30 minutes.

Open up the air fryer and carefully lay the tandoori chicken in a single layer on either the rack or in the basket of your air fryer.

Using a silicone brush, baste the chicken with either oil or ghee on one side.

Cook at 350F for 10 minutes.

Remove and flip over the chicken, and baste on the other side,

Cook for another 5 minutes.

Using a meat thermometer, check to see if the internal temperature has reached 165F. Do not skip this step.

Remove and place on a serving plate. Add lemon juice and mix, and sprinkle with cilantro.

Nutrition

- Calories: 178 kcal
- Carbohydrates: 2g

- Protein: 25g
- Fat: 6g

Crispy Chicken Nuggets

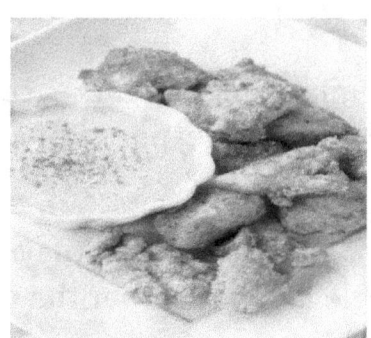

This crispy low carb chicken nuggets is quick and easy to make in the Air Fryer.

Total Time: 25 minutes

Servings 4

Ingredients

- 1 lb chicken tenders
- 1 bag pork rinds (3.25 oz)
- 1/2 cup parmesan cheese
- 1 teaspoon paprika
- 1 teaspoon garlic powder
- 1/4 cup mayo

Instructions

Pour the contents of the pork rinds in to a baggie and crush into the form of bread crumbs. Pour into a large shallow bowl and mix in the spices and cheese.

Either cut or just add the tenders to a large plastic baggie and spoon the mayo on top.

Squish the mayo and chicken around to cover the chicken completely.

Piece by piece cover the chicken with the bread crumbs and carefully place in the basket of the air fryer.

Cook for 15min at 380 degrees F and then 5 minutes at 400 degrees. Check to make sure the chicken is cooked, especially with the tenders.

Serve immediately.

Nutrition

- 389 kcal
- 24.3g fat
- 1.2g carbs
- 43.8g protein

Herb-Marinated Chicken Thighs

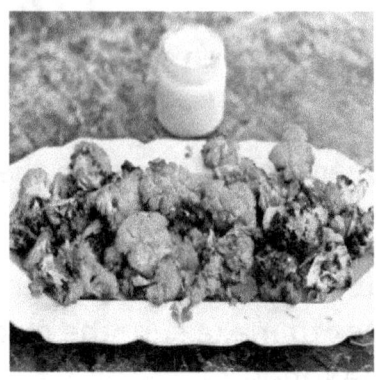

Herb-Marinated Chicken Thighs are an inexpensive, quick, and tasty idea for a low-carb breakfast.

Total time: 50 min

Serves: 8

Ingredients

- 8 bone-in, skin-on chicken thighs
- 1/4 cup olive oil
- 2 Tbs lemon juice
- 2 tsp. garlic powder
- 1 tsp. Spike Seasoning, or use any all-purpose herb blend.
- 1 tsp. dried basil
- 1/2 tsp. dried oregano
- 1/2 tsp. onion powder
- 1/2 tsp. dried sage
- 1/4 tsp. black pepper

Instructions

Cook chicken up-side down in the pre-heated air fryer for 8 minutes. Then turn the chicken thighs over and cook about 6 minutes more. After six minutes, check the chicken to see if some pieces are getting too browned and rearrange the chicken thighs in the air-fryer basket if needed. Cook about 6 minutes more, or until the chicken is well-browned with crispy skin and the internal temperature is at least 165F/75C.

Serve hot. If you want to use the air fryer and need to cook two batches for a larger family, keep the first batch warm in a 200F/100C oven while the second batch cooks.

Nutrition

- Calories: 100 kcal
- Total Fat: 9g
- Carbohydrates: 1g
- Protein: 4g

Popcorn Chicken

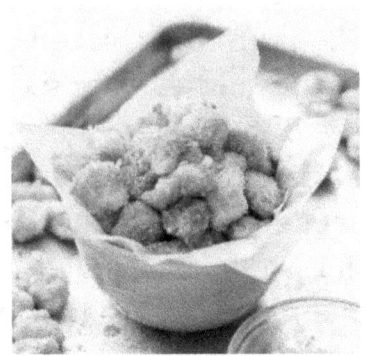

Easy and extra crunchy air fryer keto popcorn chicken that's perfect for a snack or breakfast!

Total Time: 25 minutes

Servings: 2

Ingredients

- 1.5 lb chicken breasts
- 1/4 cup coconut flour
- 1/2 tsp sea salt
- 1/4 tsp ground black pepper
- 4 eggs
- 2 1/2 cups pork panko
- 1 tsp onion powder
- 1 tsp garlic powder
- 1 tsp paprika

Instructions

In a small bowl, combine coconut flour, sea salt, and ground black pepper.

In another bowl, crack the eggs and whisk them together.

In the 3rd bowl, mix together pork panko, onion powder, garlic powder, and paprika.

Cut the chicken into bite-sized pieces, and transfer to a large mixing bowl.

Sprinkle the coconut flour mixture over the chicken and toss together gently until all of the chicken is covered evenly.

Working in batches, dredge the chicken pieces in the egg wash.

Shake off the excess and press into the pork panko mixture. Transfer to a plate and repeat with the rest of the chicken.

Lightly grease the air fryer basket, then preheat the air fryer to 400 degrees F for about 5 minutes.

Add the chicken into the air fryer basket in an even layer. If you have a small air fryer, you may need to split it up into 2 batches.

Cook for 10-12 minutes in the air fryer, shaking halfway through.

Nutrition

- Calories 263 kcal

- Fat 11g
- Carbohydrates 3g
- Protein 35g

Greek Chicken Stir-Fry

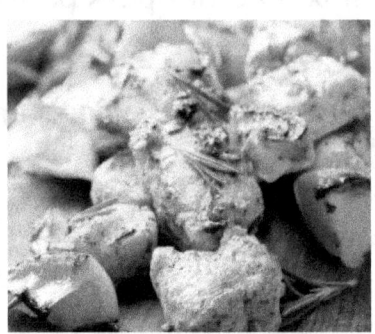

Total Time: 30 min

Serves: 2

Ingredients

- 1 (6-ounce) chicken breast, cut into 1" cubes
- 1/2 medium zucchini, chopped
- 1/2 medium red bell pepper, seeded and chopped
- 1/4 medium red onion, peeled and sliced
- 1 tablespoon coconut oil
- 1 teaspoon dried oregano
- 1/2 teaspoon garlic powder
- 1/4 teaspoon dried thyme

Instructions

Place all ingredients into a large mixing bowl and toss until the coconut oil coats the meat and vegetables. Pour the contents of the bowl into the air fryer basket.

Adjust the temperature to 375°F and set the timer for 15 minutes.

Shake the fryer basket halfway through the cooking time to redistribute the food.

Serve immediately.

Nutrition

- Calories: 186 kcal
- Fat: 8.0 g
- Protein: 20.4 g
- Carbs: 3.9 g

Parmesan Chicken Meatballs

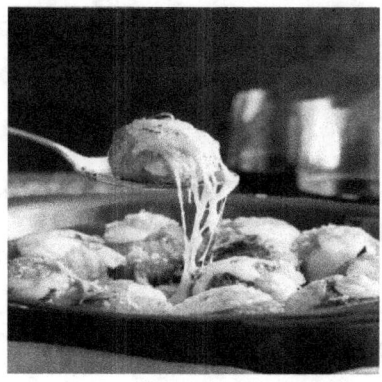

Total Time: 22 mins

Yields: 20 meatballs

A healthy recipe, that's simple to make, contains very little carbs and has a flavorful crispy crust

Ingredients

- 1 pound ground chicken
- 1 large egg, beaten
- ½ cup Parmesan cheese, grated
- ½ cup pork rinds, ground
- 1 teaspoon garlic powder
- 1 teaspoon paprika
- 1 teaspoon kosher salt
- ½ teaspoon pepper

Breading

- ½ cup pork rinds, ground

Instructions

Preheat Air Fryer to 400°F.

In a large bowl, combine chicken, egg, cheese, pork rinds (1/2 cup), garlic, paprika, salt and pepper. Roll into 1½-inch balls.

Roll the meatballs in the ground pork rinds.

Coat the air fryer basket with cooking spray, add meatballs in a single layer and cook for 12 minutes at 400°F, turning once.

Nutrition

- Calories 74.5 kcal
- Total Fat 3.6 g

- Total Carbohydrate 0.1 g
- Protein 10.1 g

6. Pork Recipes

Breakfast Sausage

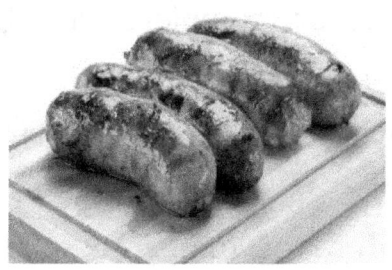

Homemade breakfast sausage has never been easier or healthier than throwing in air fryer! So delicious, easy, and freezer friendly for grab and go breakfasts.

Total Time: 20 Min

Servings: 8

Ingredients

- 1 lb ground pork
- 1 lb ground turkey
- 2 tsp fennel seeds
- 2 tsp dry rubbed sage
- 2 tsp garlic powder
- 1 tsp paprika
- 1 tsp sea salt
- 1 tsp dried thyme

- 1 tbsp real maple syrup

Instructions

Begin by mixing together the pork and turkey in a large bowl. In a small bowl, mix together the remaining ingredients: fennel, sage, garlic powder, paprika, salt, and thyme. Pour spices into the meat and continue to mix until the spices are completely incorporated.

Spoon into balls (about 2-3 tbsp of meat), and flatten into patties. Place inside the air fryer, you will probably have to do this in 2 batches.

Set the temperature to 370 degrees, and cook for 10 minutes. Remove from the air fryer and repeat with the remaining sausage.

Nutrition

- Calories: 258 kcal
- Fat: 20.5g
- Carbohydrates: 3.2g
- Protein: 14.3g.

Crispy Pork Chops

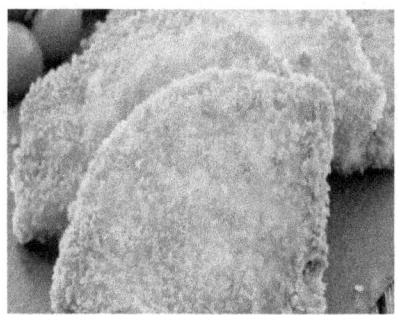

Have this recipe on the table in less then 20 minutes from start to finish. Follow the recipe as directed, or try changing it up with your favorite seasonings to make it your own.

Total Time: 17 minutes

Servings: 6 servings

Ingredients

- 1 1/2 lb boneless pork chops
- 1/3 cup Almond Flour
- 1/4 cup grated Parmesan cheese
- 1 tsp garlic powder
- 1 tsp Tony Chachere's Creole Seasoning
- 1 tsp Paprika

Instructions

Preheat your air fryer to 360 degrees F

Meanwhile, combine all ingredients EXCEPT pork chops into a large ziplock bag.

Place the pork chops into the bag, seal it, and then shake to coat the pork chops.

Remove from the bag and place in the air fryer in a single layer. Cook for 8-12 minutes depending upon the thickness of your pork chops.

Nutrition

- Calories: 231 kcal
- Carbohydrates: 2g
- Protein: 27g
- Fat: 12g

Pork Chops & Broccoli

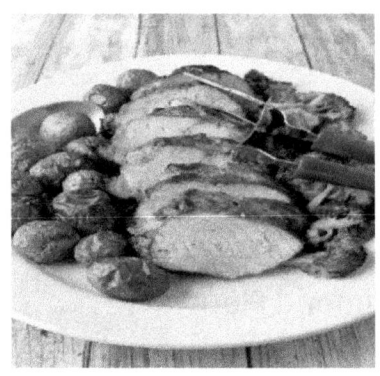

(ignore the potato in the above photo)

Total Time: 15 min

Serves: 2

Ingredients

- 2 5 ounce bone-in pork chops
- 2 tablespoons avocado oil, divided
- 1/2 teaspoon paprika
- 1/2 teaspoon onion powder
- 1/2 teaspoon garlic powder
- 1 teaspoon salt, divided
- 2 cups broccoli florets
- 2 cloves garlic, minced

Instructions

Preheat air fryer according to manufacturer's instructions to 350 degrees. Spray basket with non-stick spray.

Drizzle 1 tablespoon of oil both sides of the pork chops.

Season the pork chops on both sides with the paprika, onion powder, garlic powder, and 1/2 teaspoon of salt.

Place pork chops in the air fryer basket and cook for 5 minutes.

While pork chops are cooking, add the broccoli, garlic, remaining 1/2 teaspoon of salt, and remaining tablespoon of oil to a bowl and toss to coat.

Open the air fryer and carefully flip the pork chops.

Add the broccoli to the basket and return to the air fryer.

Cook for 5 more minutes, stirring the broccoli halfway through.

Carefully remove the food from the air fryer and serve.

Nutrition

- Calories: 483 kcal
- Total Fat: 30g
- Sugar: 2g
- Protein: 40g

Pork Chops With Brown Butter & Sage

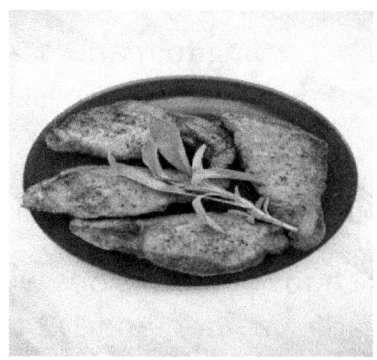

Keto pork chops made extra easy and delicious in the air fryer. Top them with brown butter and crispy sage leaves for an out-of-this-world low carb meal.

Total Time: 25 min

Servings: 4

Ingredients

- 4 medium boneless pork chops
- 6 tbsp butter divided
- Salt and pepper

- 3 tbsp chopped fresh sage

Instructions

Pat the pork chops dry. Melt one tablespoon of the butter and brush over both sides of the chops. Then sprinkle both sides with salt and pepper.

Place the chops on the air fryer rack and cook at 400F for 10 minutes. Flip the chops over and cook for another 8 to 10 minutes, until the chops register 140F on an instant read thermometer. Remove to a platter and tent with foil.

Place the remaining butter in a medium saucepan over medium heat. Let melt and then continue to cook until the butter become a rich amber brown, about 4 minutes. Watch it carefully to avoid burning.

Remove from heat and immediately add the chopped sage. It will sizzle and crisp in the hot butter.

Serve the pork chops with the browned butter and sage spooned over top.

Nutrition

- 485 kcal
- Fat 30.5g
- Carbohydrates 0.7g
- Protein 46.7g

Bacon Wrapped Jalapeno Poppers

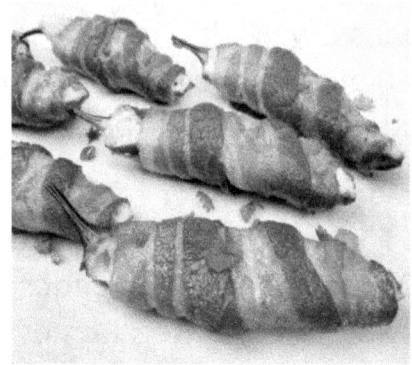

A roasted jalapeno pepper with melted cream cheese and crispy bacon!

Total Time: 24 min

Serves: 2

Ingredients

- 6 fresh jalapeno peppers
- 1/3 cup cream cheese, softened
- 6 slices of raw bacon

Directions

Slice the jalapenos in half lengthwise and remove seeds.

Fill each jalapeno slice with cream cheese using a spoon.

Cut the slices of raw bacon in half and wrap each jalapeno.

Place poppers in the air fryer and set to 370 degrees for 14 minutes.

(Note: Your cook time may vary slightly due to your thickness of bacon and pepper. It's super easy to close the machine and add a couple of minutes of cook time)

Enjoy!

Nutrition

- Calories: 180 kcal
- Total Carbohydrates: 2g
- Total Fat: 14g
- Protein: 11g

7. Other Recipes

Low Carb Zucchini Fries

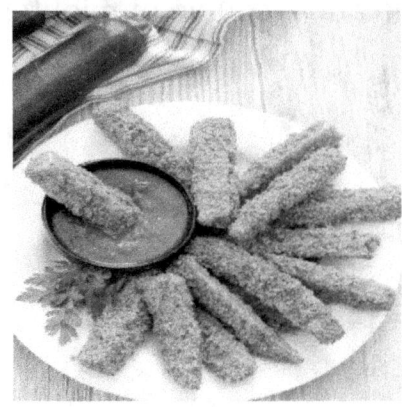

These low carb and keto friendly zucchini fries are light, crispy, and packed full of flavor at only 3 net carbs per serving in under 15 minutes!

Total Time: 15 minutes

Servings: 4

Ingredients

- 2 medium zucchini
- 1 large egg beaten
- ½ cup almond flour
- ½ cup parmesan cheese grated
- 1 teaspoon Italian seasoning or seasoning of choice
- ½ teaspoon garlic powder optional

- Pinch of salt and pepper
- Oil for spraying olive

Instructions

Cut the zucchini in half and into sticks (aka fries) about 1/2 inch thick and 3-4 inches long.

In a shallow bowl, combine the almond flour (or bread crumbs), grated parmesan, spices and a pinch of salt and pepper. Mix to combine.

Dredge zucchini in egg and then in the almond flour mixture and place on a plate or baking sheet. Generously spray zucchini with cooking spray.

Working in batches, place the zucchini fries in a single layer in the air fryer. and Cook for 10 minutes at 400F, or until crispy.

Notes

<u>Seasoning options:</u> Make these zucchini fries your own by spicing them up with your favorite seasoning mix. You can't go wrong with Italian seasoning but cajun seasoning, taco seasoning, ranch seasoning or your favorite seasoning blend will take these zucchini fries to the next level!

Nutrition

- Calories: 147 kcal
- Carbohydrates: 6g

- Protein: 9g
- Fat: 10g

Fried Cheesecake Bites

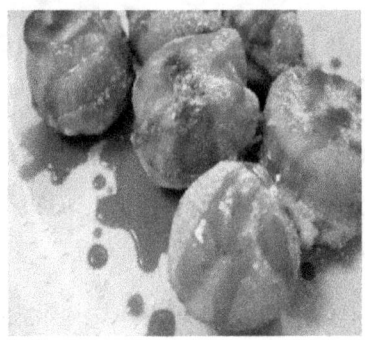

Total Time: 55 min

Yield: 16

Ingredients

- 8 ounces cream cheese
- 1/2 cup erythritol
- 4 Tablespoons heavy cream, divided
- 1/2 teaspoon vanilla extract
- 1/2 cup almond flour
- 2 Tablespoons erythritol

Instructions

Allow the cream cheese to sit on the counter for 20 minutes to soften.

Fit a stand mixer with paddle attachment.

Mix the softened cream cheese, 1/2 cup erithrytol, vanilla and heavy cream until smooth.

Scoop onto a parchment paper lined baking sheet.

Freeze for about 30 minutes, until firm.

Mix the almond flour with the 2 Tablespoons erythritol in a small mixing bowl.

Dip the frozen cheesecake bites into 2 Tablespoons cream, then roll into the almond flour mixture.

Place in an air fryer at 300 degrees for 2 minutes.

Nutrition

- Calories: 80 kcal
- Total Fat: 7g
- Carbohydrates: 2g
- Protein: 2g

Avocado Fries

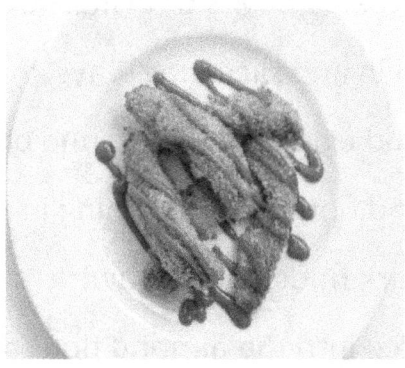

Air Fryer Avocado Fries are crispy, low in bad fat and high in the good!

Serves: 4

Total Time: 20 min

Ingredients

- 2 avocados, slightly under ripe, this makes them easier to slice
- 1/3 cup almond flour
- 1 1/2 cups pork rinds, crushed
- 2 eggs, beaten
- 2 tbsp heavy cream
- 1/2 tsp paprika
- 1/2 tsp garlic powder
- 1/2 tsp salt & pepper
- 1/4 tsp each cumin and cayenne (optional)

Instructions

Note: you will need 3 bowls or dishes for dredging

Peel avocado skin and slice long ways, evenly

Whisk cream and eggs together in one bowl

Combine almond flour and seasoning in one bowl

Add crushed pork rinds to one bowl

Dip avocado slice into the almond flour mixture coating evenly, then into the egg, then the pork rinds.

Place coated avocado slice into air fryer in a single layer.

Set air fryer at 400° for 5 minutes.

Flip avocado fries.

Set timer for 4-5 minutes. Remove.

Serve with your favorite dipping sauce or eat plain.

Nutrition

- Calories: 391 kcal
- Carbohydrates: 2.7g
- Protein: 6.1g
- Fats: 19g

Mozzarella Sticks

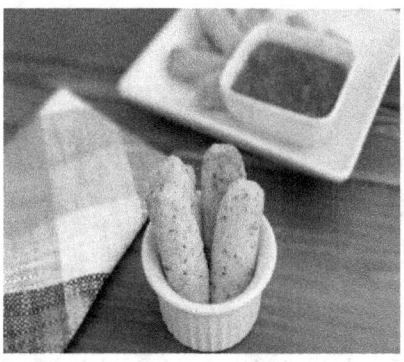

An air fryer recipe that makes amazingly crunchy, ooey-gooey fried mozzarella sticks!

Please note that this recipe requires freezing for an hour or more.

Total Time: 1hr 23 min

Serves: 4

Ingredients

- 6 mozzarella string cheese sticks (MUST be low moisture, part skim)
- 1-2 large eggs, beaten
- 1/2 cup finely grated parmesan cheese
- 1/3 cup blanched almond flour
- 1 teaspoon Italian seasoning
- 1/2 teaspoon garlic powder
- 1/4 teaspoon sea salt

Directions

If needed, prep your air fryer basket insert with a tin foil liner.

Unwrap the cheese sticks and cut in half to create two shorter sticks from each. Set aside.

Beat your egg/eggs in a small to medium bowl. You can start with one egg and add another later if needed.

In a medium dish (large enough to make it easy to coat your cheese sticks) blend together the parmesan cheese, almond flour, Italian seasoning, garlic powder, and sea salt.

Create a dipping station starting with your (previously cut) cheese sticks, followed by the egg wash, then the "breading" mix, and finally a small pan or dish covered with a sheet of parchment paper.

One by one, dip each cheese stick in the egg wash followed by rolling the cheese stick in the "breading" mix. I use a method to help adhere the "breading" to the cheese by rolling between my palms which helps to press and secure the almond flour/parmesan coating onto the cheese stick. Repeat these steps a second time before placing the fully coated cheese stick on the parchment paper. To summarize, be sure that each cheese stick gets two egg washes and two rolls in the almond flour/parmesan breading.

Once all the cheese sticks have been dipped and rolled, check each one to make sure that no cheese is showing through. Re-roll any that need extra "breading". If the cheese stick isn't fully coated then there is a greater risk that cheese will ooze out during cooking. You should have very little of the almond flour/parmesan mixture left by the time you are done with the coating process.

Place the pan/dish with cheese sticks in the freezer on a level surface for no less than 1 hour. This helps to keep the cheese from melting too quickly in the high heat of the air fryer giving the outer coating time to get crispy.

Once frozen through, remove the cheese sticks from the freezer. With cooking spray, grease your air fryer basket and/or tin foil liner as well as each cheese stick. (I spray the top side then roll them over and spray the other side.)

Place cheese sticks in air fryer. (If you have a smaller air fryer, you may want to separate into two batches as the mozzarella sticks puff a bit while cooking.) Cook at 375-400 degrees for 7-10 minutes depending on your air fryer. After 5 minutes in the air fryer, I suggest checking them every minute or so moving forward. If you see cheese start to ooze out, then it's time to pull them.

Serve immediately to ensure that your fried mozzarella sticks remain crispy, melty and gooey

Enjoy!

Additional Notes

Store leftovers in the refrigerator. Reheat in air fryer for about 5 minutes. Leftovers crisp up beautifully!

Nutrition

- Calories: 246 kcal
- Net Carbs: 2g
- Total Fat: 18g
- Protein: 19g

Delicious Rolls

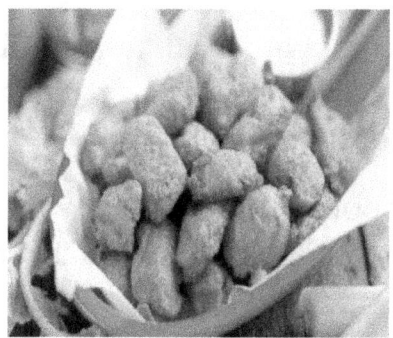

These easy keto air fryer rolls are the perfect bread substitute to support your low carb lifestyle! With only a few simple ingredients, they'll quickly become a staple.

Total Time: 20 Minutes

Serves: 2

Ingredients

- 2 cups almond flour
- 2 cups mozzarella cheese, shredded
- 2 tablespoons butter
- 1 and 1/2 teaspoons baking powder
- 1 teaspoon vinegar

For Egg Wash

- 1 egg
- 1 tablespoons butter

Instructions

In a large microwave safe bowl, combine almond flour, mozzarella cheese and butter. Microwave for 90 seconds or until cheese and butter are melted.

Mix dough together with a rubber spatula until well combined. Add baking powder and vinegar before mixing again thoroughly.

Once dough is cool enough to work with your hands, separate dough into 8 balls for rolls. Let rolls sit for 5 minutes.

Melt 2 additional tablespoons of butter in the microwave before mixing together with egg. Brush the mixture on the top of each roll.

Line your air fryer basket with parchment paper and place rolls onto parchment. You may have to work in batches depending on the size of your air fryer.

Set air fryer to 350 degrees for 10 minutes. Halfway through, use tongs to flip rolls for even cooking.

When the timer goes off, remove rolls from air fryer basket. Allow rolls to set and cool completely before eating.

Nutrition

- Calories: 296 kcal
- Total Fat: 24.5g
- Carbohydrates: 6.1g
- Protein: 14.5g

Air Fryer Biscuits

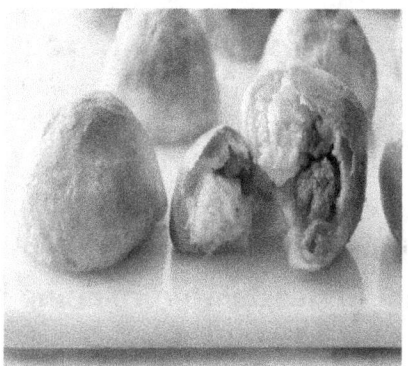

Total Time: 15 min

Servings: 9

Ingredients

- 1 cup almond flour
- 1/2 tsp baking powder
- 1/4 tsp pink himalayan salt
- 1 cup shredded cheddar cheese
- 2 large eggs
- 2 tbsp butter, melted
- 2 tbsp sour cream

Instructions

Combine the almond flour, baking powder, and salt in a large bowl. Mix in the cheddar cheese by hand until well combined.

Add eggs, butter, and sour cream to the center and blend with a large fork, spoon, or your hands, until a sticky batter forms.

Fit a piece of parchment paper into your air fryer basket. Drop ¼ cup-sized (for large) or 2 tablespoon-sized (for small) portions of batter onto the parchment.

Air Fry/"Bake" at 400 degrees F for 6 minutes (for small) to 10 minutes (for large), until golden brown and cooked through. Repeat with remaining batter as needed. Serve immediately!

Note: recipe can yield 9 small biscuits or 5 large biscuits.

Nutrition is for 9 small biscuits.

Alternatively, you could place the batter in silicone muffin liners and air fry them for taller biscuits (yields 7-9, bakes 10-12 minutes depending on how much you fill them).

Nutrition

- Calories 167 kcal
- Fat 15g
- Carbohydrates 3g
- Protein 7g

Air Fry Olive Bread

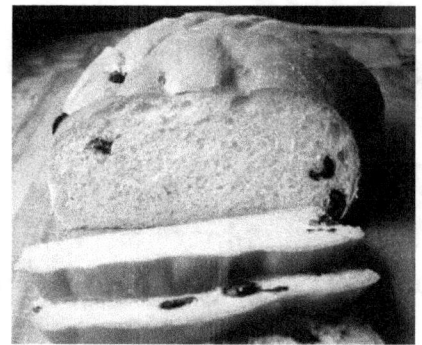

Cook Time: 30 minutes

Servings: 6

Ingredients

- 1 cup + 2 table spoon Almond Flour
- 1 tsp Baking Powder
- 1/4 tsp Salt
- 1/4 tsp Baking Soda
- 1 tsp Monk Fruit Sweetener granules
- 1/4 cup Flaxseed Meal
- 1 large Egg
- tablespoons olive oil
- 1/3 cup Black Olives chopped coarsly
- 1 tablespoon Water

Instructions

Prepare an Air Fryer cooking pan with cooking spray so the bread dough does not stick.

In a large bowl mix all the ingredients together until well combined.

Shape the dough into a round loaf (or shape of choice) and put it inside the pan. Place the pan inside the Air Fryer and cook on the bread/cake setting. (Should be 330 degrees for about 30 minutes on the Air Fryer, some temps may vary)

Cook the bread until the timer goes off. The bread should rise a bit and be completely dry on the top and bottom of the loaf. (If not you can cook a bit longer)

Nutrition

- Calories 256 kcal
- Fat 23.6g
- Protein 6.4 g
- Net Carbs 2.4 g

Lunch & Dinner Recipes

1. Chicken Recipes

Chicken Thighs With Adobo Seasoning

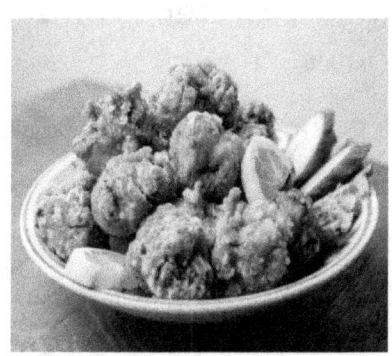

Delicious air fried chicken thighs with a crispy, crunchy adobo seasoning crust that is naturally low carb and bursting with flavor!

Total time: 25 min

Serves: 4

Ingredients

- 4 large chicken thighs
- 2 tbsp adobo seasoning (Use Light or Low Sodium Adobo seasoning if you like chicken less salty)
- 1 tbsp olive oil

Instructions

Add olive oil to bag or plate and coat chicken in it.

Toss chicken thighs in adobo seasoning to coat.

Place chicken thighs in air fryer basket, making sure they don't touch or crowd each other.

Set air fryer to 350 degrees and set the timer to 10 minutes.

After 10 minutes, flip chicken to other side and cook another 10 minutes.

Chicken will be golden brown and 165 degrees internal temperature at the end of cooking.

Nutrition

- Calories: 340 kcal
- Carbs: 2g
- Fats: 14g
- Protein: 26g

Buttermilk Fried Chicken

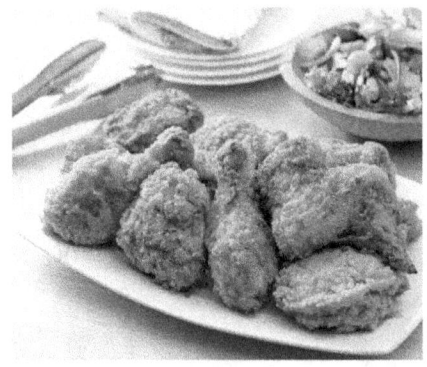

This awesome recipe is a traditional, Southern soul food recipe. This dish is quick to whip up, with less than

7 ingredients. The results are crispy, crunchy fried wings.

Total Time: 30 minutes

Servings: 5

Ingredients

- 2 1/2-3 pounds whole chicken wings
- 1/4 cup buttermilk
- 3/4 cup almond flour
- McCormick's Grill Mates Montreal Chicken seasoning, to taste
- salt and pepper to taste
- cooking oil

Instructions

Add the chicken wings to a large bowl. Drizzle with the buttermilk.

Combine almond flour, chicken seasoning, salt and pepper in a bowl large enough to dredge the chicken. Stir and mix well.

Dredge the chicken in the flour and seasonings. Ensure both sides of the chicken are fully coated. Use a spoon to get areas of the chicken wing that were missed.

Spray the air fryer basket with cooking oil.

Add the chicken wings to the air fryer. It's ok to stack the chicken, but do not overcrowd the basket. Cook in batches if necessary

Cook for 20 minutes on 400 degrees. Stop and flip the chicken every 5 minutes, a total of 4 times.

Ensure the chicken is cooked on the inside. Use a meat thermometer and ensure the chicken has reached an internal temperature of 160 degrees. Add additional time if you prefer the chicken is crisper.

Remove from the air fryer. Cool before serving.

Nutrition

- Calories: 240 kcal
- fats: 14g
- sugars: 0.5g
- protein: 18g

Gochujang Chicken Wings (Korean Recipe)

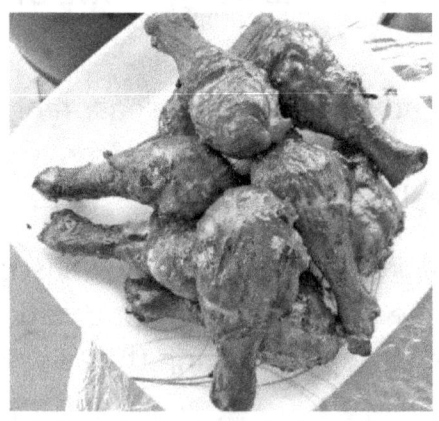

This recipe make a delightful easy keto appetizer or meal. Make it in your air fryer and enjoy the finger-licking goodness.

Total Time: 40 minutes

Servings: 4

Ingredients

For the Wings:

- 2 pounds chicken wings
- 1 teaspoon Salt
- 1 teaspoon Ground Black Pepper, or gochujaru

For the Sauce:

- 2 tablespoons gochujang
- 1 tablespoon mayonnaise
- 1 teaspoon agave nectar
- 1 tablespoon Sesame Oil
- 1 tablespoon minced ginger
- 1 tablespoon Minced Garlic
- 1/3 cup stevia

For Finishing:

- 2 teaspoons Sesame Seeds, optional
- 1/4 cup Green Onions, optional

Instructions

Preheat your air fryer to 400°F

Salt and Pepper the chicken wings and place in the air fryer basket.

Set the timer to 20 minutes and allow the chicken wings to cook, turning once at 10 minutes.

As the chicken bakes or air fries, mix together all the sauce ingredients and let the sauce marinate while the chicken wings finish cooking.

As you near the 20-minute mark use a thermometer to check the meat. When the chicken wings reach 160F remove them from the oven and place into a bowl.

Pour about half the sauce on the wings, and toss to coat the wings with the sauce.

Place the chicken wings back into the oven or air fryer and cook for another 5 minutes until the sauce has glazed over, and the chicken is completely cooked and has reached at least 165F.

Remove, sprinkle with sesame seeds and chopped green onions and serve!

Nutrition

- Calories: 356 kcal
- Carbohydrates: 6g
- Protein: 23g
- Fat: 26g

Chicken Wings With Sauce

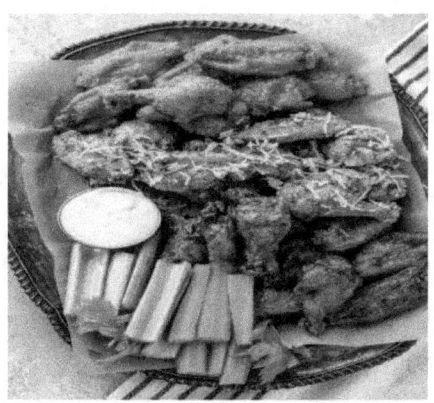

You will not believe how easy and crispy these air fryer chicken wings are! They are ready in under 30 minutes, perfectly crispy, and the clean up is so easy!

Total Time: 27 minutes

Servings: 2

Ingredients For Chicken Wings

- 1 Tablespoon Extra Virgin Olive Oil
- 4 Pounds Fresh Chicken Wings
- Salt and Pepper to taste

Ingredients For Chicken Wing Sauce

Yield: 8 quarter-litre jars

- 10 cups of tomatoes washed, peeled, cored and chopped
- 2 cups onions chopped.

- 1/2 teaspoon liquid stevia
- 1/2 teaspoon cayenne pepper
- 12 oz white vinegar (5% or higher)
- 4 teaspoons salt
- 2 cloves garlic , minced
- 1 teaspoon allspice ground
- 1 teaspoon cinnamon ground
- 1 teaspoon cloves ground
- 1 teaspoon ginger

Instructions For Chicken Wing Sauce

Prepare the tomatoes.

Put into a large pot (at least 4 litres / quart).

Peel and chop the onion. Add to pot.

Add the stevia and the cayenne. Bring to a boil uncovered.

Lower to a gentle boil and let simmer uncovered until onion has softened -- about 30 minutes.

Remove from heat, let cool a bit.

Purée in batches in a blender or food processor.

Return mixture to pot.

Add all the remaining ingredients from the vinegar downwards. Bring to a boil.

Reduce to a simmer and let simmer uncovered until the consistency of a somewhat thin ketchup -- about an hour.

Ladle sauce into heated jars, leaving 2 cm (1/2 inch) headspace. Debubble, adjust headspace.

Wipe jar rims. Put lids on.

Process in a water bath or steam canner.

Process jars for 15 minutes; increase time as needed for your altitude

Instructions – Chicken Wings

Using a paper towel, oil the inside of the air fryer with the oil.

Pat the chicken wings dry with paper towels. Season with salt and pepper

Place the chicken wings inside the Air Fryer basket.

Set the Air Fryer temperature to 380F and the time for 25 minutes. Cook the chicken wings in the Air Fryer, removing the basket every 5 minutes to toss for even cooking.

After the 25 minutes are up, toss the chicken wings one more time and finish cooking. Increase the temperature to 400F and cook for 5 more minutes.

Serve immediately or coat in your favorite wing sauce.

Nutrition

- Calories: 430 kcal
- Protein 25g
- Carbs: 3g

- Fats: 12g

4-Ingredients Keto Wings

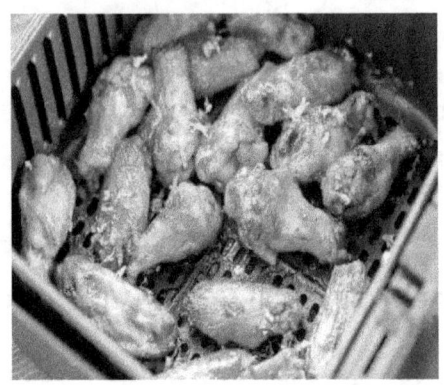

Make crispy, crowd-pleasing wings in the air fryer with very little effort!

Serves: 4

Total Time: 37 min

Ingredients

- 12 chicken wings, uncooked
- salt & pepper to taste
- 1 tablespoon olive oil spray
- 3 tablespoons buffalo chicken wing sauce

Directions

Simply place raw chicken wings in air fryer basket. Salt & pepper to taste. Mist with cooking spray.

SET THE TIMER FOR 30 MINUTES AT 370 DEGREES FAHRENHEIT.

At the halfway mark, turn them and mist the wings with cooking spray.

Once they are done cooking to your desired crispness, toss with wing sauce and enjoy!

Note: Refer to the next recipe (on page 103) for the buffalo sauce recipe!

Nutrition

- Calories: 273 kcal
- Total Carbohydrates:0g
- Total Fat: 20g
- Protein: 22g

Chicken Hot Wings With Buffalo Sauce

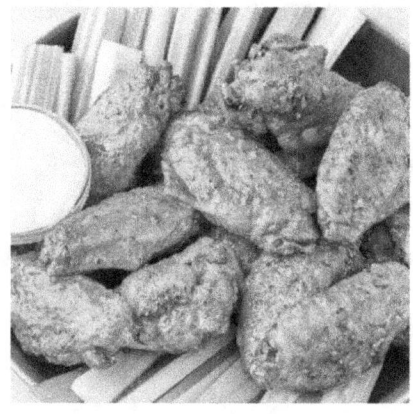

Got a craving for buffalo wings but don't have time to head out to a pub or restaurant? Make them in your air fryer. It'll take less than 35 minutes to make the recipe.

Total Time: 34 minutes

Servings: 5 people

Ingredients

Wings:

- 2 pounds chicken wingettes
- 1 tablespoon olive oil or avocado oil
- 1/2 teaspoon garlic powder
- 1/2 teaspoon salt
- extra oil for greasing

Buffalo Sauce:

- 1/3 cup hot pepper sauce (You can use Frank's Red Hot)
- 1/4 cup butter butter flavored coconut oil for dairy-free
- 1 tablespoon white vinegar
- 1/8 teaspoon ground chipolte pepper or cayenne pepper

Instructions

For the Buffalo Sauce:

While wings are cooking in air fryer, combine hot sauce, butter, vinegar, and ground pepper in small pot.

Bring sauce to a boil on medium heat while whisking everything together. Remove from heat and set aside.

When wings are done, add them to the sauce and coat each piece evenly.

Serve with blue cheese dressing and celery.

Wings:

In large bowl, rub olive oil on chicken wings and then sprinkle on the garlic powder and salt.

Rub inside of air fryer basket with a little more olive oil, avocado oil, or coconut oil.

Place chicken wings in a single layer in basket.

Cook wings at 360°F for 25 minutes.

Flip wings over. Then increase temperature to 400°F and cook for 4 more minutes.

Nutrition

- Calories: 327 kcal
- Carbohydrates: 0g
- Protein: 18g
- Fat: 27g

Whole Chicken Recipe

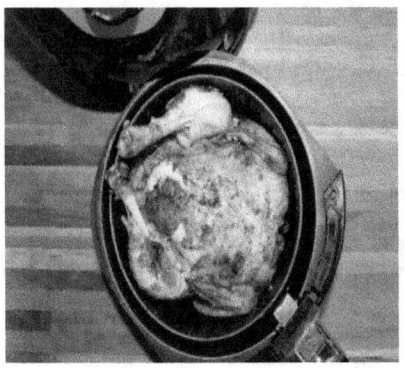

Total time: 1hr

servings: 4

Ingredients

For a 5 qt. Air fryer:

- 3 lbs whole chicken
- 1.5 tsp coarse salt
- ¼ tsp each black pepper, sweet paprika
- ½ tsp each garlic, onion powder,
- ½ tsp each dry rosemary, dry thyme (or 1 tsp Italian seasoning)

For a 6 qt. Air fryer:

- 4 lbs whole chicken
- 2 tsp coarse salt
- 1/4 tsp each black pepper, sweet paprika
- ½ tsp each garlic, onion powder

- ½ tsp each dry rosemary, dry thyme (or 1 tsp Italian seasoning)

Directions

Remove the giblets inside the whole chicken cavity. Pat dry with a clean paper towel.

Combine dry spice seasonings from salt to thyme in a bowl.

Use your fingers to gently separate the skin from the meat to create small pockets. Be careful not to tear the skin. Stuff the dry spice mixture under the skin and use your hands to gently spread the spices as even as you can. Make sure to season the outer interior and the back of the bird.

Place the whole chicken breast side down in the air fryer. Roast at 360F for 30 minutes.

Flip the chicken (now breast side up and roast at the same temperature for 20 minutes (3 lbs. chicken) or 25 minutes (4 lbs. chicken).

Test the internal temperature with a meat thermometer. It should reach at least 165F at the thickest part without touching the bones. If not, send it back and roast for 5 additional minutes then test the temperature again.

Allow the chicken to rest for 10 minutes before carving. The bottom of the air fryer basket will catch all the chicken juice. Serve the juice on the side if you like.

Nutrition

- calories: 356 kcal
- carbohydrates: 1g
- protein: 31g
- fat: 25g

Spicy Dry-Rubbed Chicken Wings

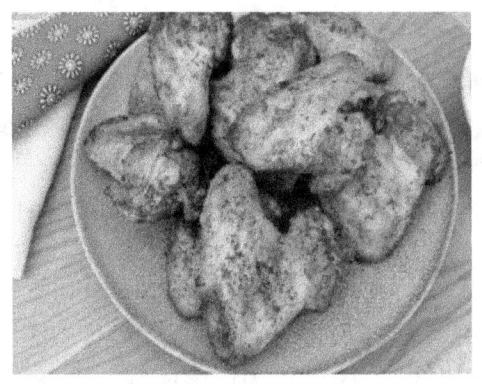

Total Time: 55 minutes

Servings: 4

Ingredients

- 2 lbs Chicken Wings

Spicy Dry Rub Ingredients

✓ 2 tbsp smoked paprika

✓ 3 tsp cayenne pepper (optional)

✓ 2 tsp chili powder

- ✓ 1 tbsp black pepper
- ✓ 1.5 tbsp garlic powder
- ✓ 2 tsp onion powder
- ✓ 1.5 tbsp Sea Salt
- ✓ 1.5 tsp Italian Seasoning
- ✓ 1.5 tsp dried thyme

Instructions

To Marinate the Wings: Place chicken in a ziploc bag with 1/4 cup of the spicy dry rub. You can store the rest in a mason jar. Shake the bag so that the mix coats the chicken evenly.Store in the refrigerator for at least four hours, ideally overnight

Next, place the chicken wings in the air fryer basket

Cook for 15 minutes per side.

Nutrition Facts

- Calories 206 kcal
- Fat 14g
- Carbohydrates 5g
- Protein 16g

Cornish Hens Recipe

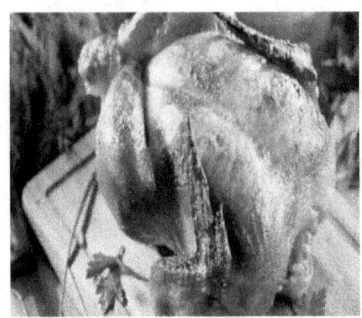

Air Fryer Cornish Hens is a gourmet dinner, straight out of the Air Fryer! Crispy outside and tender and juicy inside makes this the perfect recipe for those fancier family gatherings or just a weekday meal!

Total Time: 50 minutes

Servings: 4

Ingredients

- 2 Cornish Game Hens
- 2 Tablespoons Avocado oil
- 1 Tablespoon kosher salt
- 1 teaspoon Ground black pepper
- 1 teaspoon garlic powder
- 1 teaspoon smoked paprika
- 1/2 teaspoon dried Basil
- 1/2 teaspoon dried Oregano
- 1/2 teaspoon dried Thyme

Instructions

Spray the inside of the air fryer with cooking spray.

Combine the avocado oil, and all of the seasongs in a small bowl.

Rub the seasoning evenly over both hens. You can even lift up the breast skin and rub some seasoning directly on the breast meat for even more flavor.

Place in the air fryer breast-side down and cook at 360F for 35 minutes.

Flip the hens and cook for an additional 10 minutes to get the skin crispy.

The hens are finished when the internal temperature is 165F.

Nutrition

- Calories: 400 kcal
- Carbohydrates: 1g
- Protein: 29g
- Fat: 31g

Almond Flour Air Fried Chicken

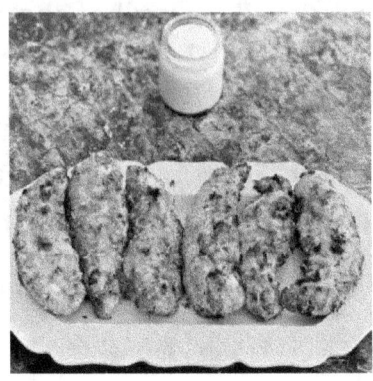

Almond Flour Air Fried Chicken is an easy low carb, gluten free and keto friendly crispy chicken recipe.

Total Time: 22 minutes

Servings: 4

Ingredients

- 4 Chicken Breasts, about 4 ounces each and pounded to an even thickness. About 1/3 inch is thickness is best.
- 1 cup Almond Flour
- 1/2 cup Parmesan Cheese
- 1 tsp. Garlic Powder
- 1 tsp. Onion Powder
- 1 tsp. Paprika
- 2 tsp. salt
- 1 tsp. pepper
- 1 egg beaten

Instructions

Trim and pound the chicken breasts. A thickness of 1/3 of an inch is best.

Salt and pepper the outside of the chicken and set aside.

Mix the egg up in a dish. Be sure it's one your chicken will fit into as you'll be dipping the chicken in the egg first.

In another dish mix together almond flour, parmesan cheese, garlic powder, onion powder, paprika, salt and pepper.

Dredge the chicken in the egg and then the almond flour mixture.

Preheat your air fryer to 390 degrees. Just allow it to run for 2-3 minutes.

Spray the air fryer basket with cooking spray. Add the chicken, then spray the tops of the chicken with cooking spray as well.

Air fry for 10-12 minutes or until the chicken reaches an internal temperature of 165 degrees. Flip it halfway through cooking. I like to use an instant read thermometer to check my chicken. It's easy to overcook it when air frying.

Nutrition

- Calories 248 kcal

- Fat 11.3g
- Carbohydrates 5g
- Protein 33g

Garlic Parmesan Chicken Wings

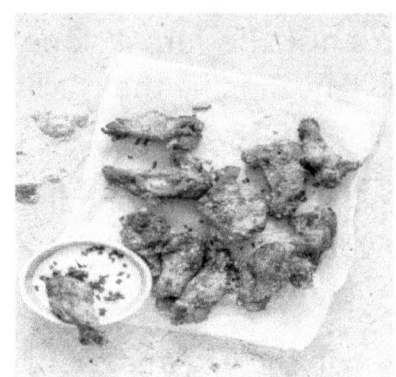

Total Time: 25 min

Serves: 6

Ingredients

- 2 pounds chicken wings (or drumsticks)
- 3/4 cup grated Parmesan cheese
- 2 teaspoons minced garlic
- 2 teaspoons fresh parsley (chopped)
- 1 teaspoon salt
- 1 teaspoon pepper

Instructions

Preheat your air fryer to 400 degrees for 3-4 minutes

Pat chicken pieces dry with a paper towel.

Mix Parmesan cheese, garlic, parsley, salt, and pepper together in a bowl.

Toss chicken pieces in cheese mixture until coated.

Place chicken in bottom of air fryer basket and set timer to 10-12 minutes.

After 12 minutes, use tongs to flip chicken.

Fry again for 12 minutes.

Remove chicken from basket with tongs and sprinkle with more Parmesan cheese and parsley.

Serve with your favorite dipping sauce.

Nutrition

- Calories 322 kcal
- Fat 23g
- Sugar 2g
- Protein 14g

Lemon-Garlic Chicken Thighs

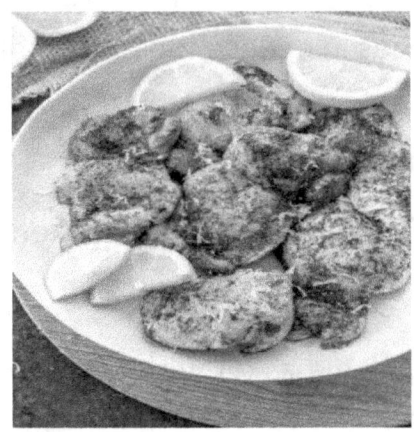

Total Time: 2 hrs 35 mins

Servings: 4

Ingredients

- ¼ cup lemon juice
- 2 tablespoons olive oil
- 1 teaspoon Dijon mustard
- 2 cloves garlic, minced
- ¼ teaspoon salt
- ⅛ teaspoon ground black pepper
- 4 skin-on, bone-in chicken thighs
- 4 lemon wedges

Directions

Whisk lemon juice, olive oil, Dijon mustard, garlic, salt, and pepper together in a bowl. Set marinade aside.

Place chicken thighs into a large resealable plastic bag. Pour marinade over chicken and seal bag, making sure to cover all parts of chicken. Refrigerate for at least 2 hours.

Preheat an air fryer to 360 degrees F (175 degrees C).

Remove chicken from marinade and pat dry with paper towels. Place chicken pieces in the air fryer basket, cooking in batches if necessary.

Fry until chicken is no longer pink at the bone and the juices run clear, 22 to 24 minutes. An instant-read thermometer inserted near the bone should read 165 degrees F (74 degrees C). Squeeze a lemon wedge over each piece upon serving.

Nutrition

- Calories: 258 kcal
- Total Fat: 18.6g
- Carbohydrates: 3.6g
- Protein: 19.4g

Chicken & Broccoli

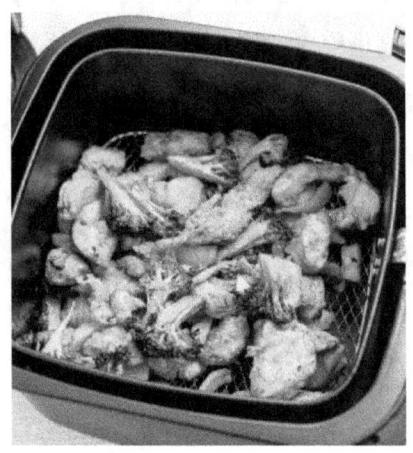

Total Time: 35 min

Servings: 4

Ingredients

- 1 pound boneless skinless chicken breast , cut into bite sized pieces
- 1/4-1/2 pound broccoli , cut into small florets (1-2 cups)
- 1/2 medium onion, sliced
- 1 Tablespoon olive oil or grape seed oil
- 1/2 teaspoon garlic powder
- 1 Tablespoon fresh minced ginger
- 1 Tablespoon low sodium soy sauce, or to taste (use Tamari for Gluten Free)
- 1 teaspoon sesame seed oil

- 2 teaspoons rice vinegar (use distilled white vinegar for Gluten Free)
- 2 teaspoons hot sauce (optional)
- additional salt, to taste
- additional black pepper, to taste
- serve with lemon wedges

Directions

In a large bowl, combine chicken breast, broccoli and onion. Toss ingredients together.

Make the Marinade: In a bowl, combine oil, garlic powder, ginger, soy sauce, sesame oil, rice vinegar and hot sauce. Pour marinade evenly over chicken/broccoli/onion in the bowl. Stir thoroughly to combine marinade over chicken, broccoli and onions.
Air Fry: Add ingredients to air fry basket. Air fry 380°F for 16-20 minutes, shaking and gently tossing halfway through cooking. Make sure to toss so that everything cooks evenly.

Check chicken to make sure it's cooked through. If not, cook for additional 3-5 minutes.

Add additional salt and pepper, to taste. Squeeze fresh lemon juice on top and serve warm.

Nutrition

- Calories 191 kcal
- Fat: 7g
- Carbohydrates: 4g

- Protein: 25g

Southern-Style Chicken Recipe

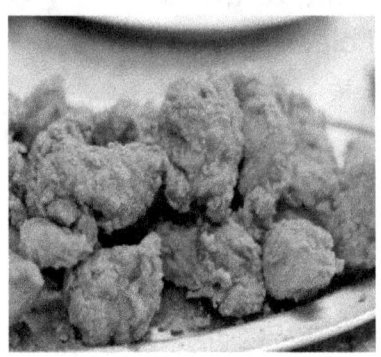

Total Time: 35 min
Serves: 6

Ingredients

- 2 cups crushed Ritz crackers (about 50)
- 1 tablespoon minced fresh parsley
- 1 teaspoon garlic salt
- 1 teaspoon paprika
- 1/2 teaspoon pepper
- 1/4 teaspoon ground cumin
- 1/4 teaspoon rubbed sage
- 1 large egg, beaten
- 1 broiler/fryer chicken (3 to 4 pounds), cut up

Directions

Preheat air fryer to 375°. Spritz the fryer basket with cooking spray.

In a shallow bowl, mix the next 7 ingredients. Place egg in a separate shallow bowl. Dip chicken in egg, then in cracker mixture, patting to help coating adhere. Place a few pieces of chicken in a single layer in the prepared basket, spritz with cooking spray.

Cook 10 minutes. Turn chicken and spritz with additional cooking spray; cook until chicken is golden brown and juices run clear, 10-20 minutes longer. Repeat with remaining chicken.

Nutrition

- 410 kcal
- 23g fat
- 2g sugars
- 36g protein.

5 – Ingredient Crispy & Cheesy Dinner Chicken

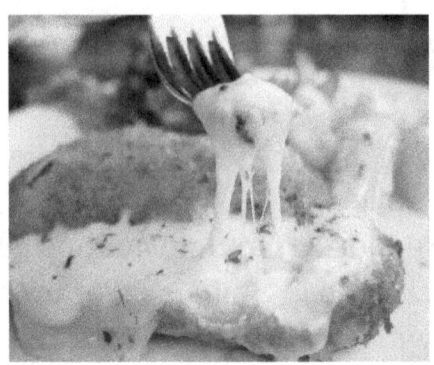

Total Time: 17 min

Serves: 4

Ingredients

- 4 thin chicken breasts (or two chicken breasts cut/pounded to be thin)
- 1 cup milk
- 1/2 cup panko bread crumbs
- 3/4-1 cup shaved Parmesan-Asiago cheese blend (can use any type of hard shaved or shredded cheese like Parmesan, Asiago, Romano)
- salt + pepper to taste

Instructions

Preheat your air fryer to 400 degrees. Spray the cooking basket lightly with cooking spray.

In a large bowl place the milk and chicken breasts. Sprinkle in a generous pinch of salt and freshly ground pepper. Allow to marinate in the milk for 10 minutes.

In a shallow bowl combine panko bread crumbs and shaved cheese.

Dredge chicken breasts through panko and cheese mixture (press the mixture on top of the chicken generously) and place in the air fryer basket. Make sure that the basket is not overcrowded. You can fit 2 chicken breasts in the basket, I did this in two batches. Spray the top of the chicken lightly with cooking spray (this 'locks on' the cheesy bread crumb topping).

Cook for 8 minutes, flipping the chicken breasts halfway through.

Remove from the air fryer, repeat the process with any remaining chicken breasts. If you want to warm everything, you can add the already cooked chicken breasts into the basket and cook them for 1 minute to warm them! Enjoy

Nutrition

- 410 kcal
- 23g fat
- 3g sugars
- 36g protein.

Pizza Stuffed Chicken

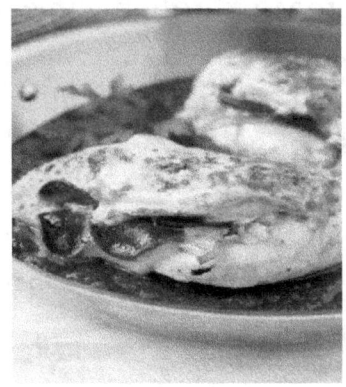

Total Time: 25 minutes

Servings 2 -3

Ingredients

- 5 boneless skinless, chicken thighs
- 1/2 cup pizza sauce (check recipe below)
- 14 slices turkey pepperoni
- 1/2 small red onion sliced
- 5 oz sliced mozzarella cheese
- 1/2 cup shredded cheese for topping

Pizza Sauce: Ingredients

- 28 oz can San Marzano peeled tomatoes
- 3 tbsp olive oil
- 2 tbsp apple cider vinegar
- 2 tsp dried basil
- 2 tsp oregano
- 1 tsp garlic powder

- 1 tsp onion powder
- 1 tsp parsley
- 1 tsp salt
- 1/2 tsp red pepper flakes
- 1/4 tsp pepper

How To Make Pizza Sauce: Instructions

In a blender, blend all ingredients together until mixture forms a sauce.

Serve on your favorite low-carb pizza crust or enjoy with other dishes that use pizza sauce.

Directions: Pizza Stuffed Chicken

Open your chicken thighs and lay them flat on a piece of parchment paper.

Place a second piece of parchment paper over the chicken.

Pound the chicken to create a thin piece. This makes the chicken easier to fold, and cook quickly. Spoon on a tablespoon of pizza sauce on each piece of chicken and spread it evenly.

Place 3 pieces of turkey pepperoni on top of the sauce.

Add one slice of Mozzarella cheese.

Fold one side of the chicken over on to the other

Use a toothpick or skewer stick to hold the chicken together. Once cooked it stays together on it's own.

Preheat the air fryer at 370F for 2 minutes. Grease the tray, and lay the pieces out in a single layer.

Add the chicken and let cook for 6 minutes. Flip and cook for another 6 minutes.

For the last 3 minutes, add cheese to melt on the top. Cooktime may vary depending on how thick your chicken pieces are. Always check chicken thighs to ensure they are heated to 165F.

Nutrition

- Calories: 282 kcal
- Carbohydrates: 4g
- Protein: 32g
- Fat: 18g

Conclusion

Air fryers make it easier to find foods you love on a low-carb or keto diet. They allow you to prepare low-carb fried foods, cook at home more easily, and explore versatile cooking options.

www.ingramcontent.com/pod-product-compliance
Lightning Source LLC
Chambersburg PA
CBHW071832080526
44589CB00012B/990